DISEASES of the DRxUGS

Christie Fleetwood, ND, RPh, FNMI, cBC

Copyright © 2026, Christie Fleetwood

All rights reserved. No part of this book may be reproduced in any form, except as applied to brief quotations incorporated into critical articles or reviews.

This book is not intended as a substitute for the medical advice of physicians. The reader should regularly consult a physician in matters relating to his/her health and particularly with respect to any symptoms that may require diagnosis or medical attention. **Do NOT take yourself off your prescription medications!**

Editors: Pamela Cangioli and Kimberley Jace
Cover and Interior Design: Creative Publishing Book Design

ISBN Paperback: 979-8-9948796-0-3
ISBN eBook: 979-8-9948796-1-0

Table of Contents

Before we begin ... v
    Assumptions ... v
    World Views ... vi
    Recognized personal biases and noteworthy beliefs ... x
    What's Coming Up In this Book? ... xii

Chapter 1: Hypertension ... 1
    Drugs that can cause hypertension ... 2
    The secondary diagnoses… ... 4
    Self-assessment ... 7
    Nutritional deficiencies ... 7
    Other interesting facts ... 9
    The case for calcium ... 9
    Other ingredients ... 10

Chapter 2: Dyslipidemia ... 15
    Drugs that can cause dyslipidemia ... 15
    Costs to consider ... 17
    The secondary diagnoses… ... 19
    Nutritional deficiencies ... 20
    Other ingredients ... 23
    Healthy snack options ... 24

Chapter 3: Type 2 diabetes ... 25
    Drugs that can cause type 2 diabetes ... 25
    The secondary diagnoses… ... 26
    Nutritional deficiencies ... 31
    Other ingredients ... 32

Appendix A: Hypertension ... 35
    Table 1 ... 36

Table 2	44
Table 3	49
Table 4	53
Rolling Blood Pressure Log	66
Appendix B: Dyslipidemia	67
Table 1	68
Table 2	73
Table 3	76
Table 4	80
Appendix C: Type 2 diabetes	85
Table 1	86
Table 2	89
Table 3	92
Table 4	93
Rolling Blood Glucose Log	98

Before We Begin...

In case no one has told you this today, *your life matters*. You know this on some level because this book is now in your hands. You're sick and tired of being sick and tired. You want to improve your health. Together, we'll work to help you take that step toward prolonging your years and giving you a better quality of life.

Before we begin this adventure together, there are assumptions, worldviews, and biases we need to tackle to help you make the most of each choice every day, as well as making the most of this two-in-one book.

Assumptions

When I set out to write this book, I made an "assumption" that you were a particular type of reader: either someone with one or more of the cardiometabolic conditions mentioned in the sub-title of this book, or a caregiver (including doctors, nurses, pharmacists, their students, and educated lay persons) caring for patients with one or more of those cardiometabolic conditions.

Here's another assumption this book makes: Satisfied readers of this book will be equally unsatisfied with the status quo in conventional medicine and the management of cardiovascular and cardiometabolic conditions. That means you likely fall into one of the following categories:

- A healthcare provider who realizes the System (of "healthcare") is broken. You see it as a disease-management system unconcerned with whole-body preventive health. You signed up to be part of the solution, but you feel like maybe you've become part of a bigger problem. Therefore, you're reading this book to find other answers, even if they're "alternative." (See my comment on this term under Biases.)
- A patient who is stuck in the broken system of disease management, sick and tired of being "managed." You have a sense that maybe, just maybe, the drug you were given to lower your blood pressure is causing the "need" for the drug to lower your cholesterol. And recently you learned that the statin-manufacturer for the cholesterol-reducing drug you're taking is being sued for pushing people into type 2 diabetes prematurely. (As if they would have become type 2 diabetics later on without the statin? Is that **an admission** that type 2 diabetes is a lifestyle-driven disease? Huh!)

- Maybe you're not quite in either of the above categories but potentially a disillusioned student of medicine or a disenfranchised consumer of conventional medicine, unwilling to become a "patient." You've likely already "failed" (or been failed by) conventional medicine. The prescription drugs make you feel worse without really moving the numbers or your symptoms in any positive direction. Medicine either hurt you or scared you sufficiently so as to have lost your trust in it.

I get it. I've been in all three categories, myself, and I've worked with countless others through similar experiences. I was a pharmacist who got radically ill, and the medicine I'd known all my life and had chosen as a career failed me. Through self-study, I educated myself and changed my lifestyle. I slowed down so I could really *hear* and bear witness to the stories of my pharmacy customers. Before long, I started asking questions that my colleagues and medical doctor friends couldn't sufficiently answer. Then I went back to school full-time to learn the things humankind had been using merely a hundred years ago to keep ourselves *well*, rather than manage what's *wrong*.

I'll also make the positive assumption that you will appreciate the conventional medical information—*all* of it including the good, the bad, the "ugly" (*Boxed Warnings*) and even the unknowns. This book is designed to provide information necessary for *informed consent* to those writing the prescriptions, those filling the prescriptions, and those taking the prescriptions.

Worldviews

Perhaps "Medical Paradigms" would be an even better header for this section. The professional association to which I belong has this on their website (I added the italicized "worldview" explanation):

MEDICAL PARADIGMS

Conventional MDs, DOs, many NDs and DCs

1. There are entities called diseases. They number about 18,000, and are given names, such as measles, lupus, DCIS, schizophrenia, etc. These entities are labeled as the **cause** of ill health and the reason people seek the help of a physician. *(Kill the bugs; correct the snps.)*

2. These disease entities can be identified through the art and science of **diagnosis**. *(Correct diagnosis is paramount as it allows for correct drug/procedure selection and protocol.)*

3. These disease entities can be **treated and eliminated**, thereby restoring the person to a state of health (more accurately stated as the absence of signs/symptoms, ie symptom control/disease management).

4. The appropriate treatment of these diseases is the **evidence-based application of, primarily, pharmaceuticals** and/or surgeries and other interventions. *(Pharmaceutical companies are for-profit businesses, primarily interested in making money!)*

Vitalist NDs, some DCs

1. The Universe is **ordered and intelligent** as is evident at the most minute levels of anatomy, physiology, chemistry and biology, and the order and intelligence we see in the body reflects the order we see in the universe. *(Symptoms are the body's wise vocabulary, speaking wisdom in the kindest way that will still get our attention to make changes in life.)*

2. **Health is the natural state of humanity**, with illness being a temporary adaptive response to disturbances in function. *(The patient's vitality is more important than the diagnosis.)*

3. **Correction of the disturbance should result in the return of the normal healthy state.** *(Use supportive measures for function/physiology. Find/treat the cause while providing individual, whole-person care.)*

4. Interventions should involve the **least force necessary** to accomplish this. *(With an emphasis on removing obstacles to cure and (re)establishing the determinants of health: namely, real food, clean water, fun movement, restorative sleep, fulfilling work, healthy relationships.)*

https://www.naturopathicmedicineinstitute.org/about/vitalism/

Before We Begin...

What does this *mean*, though? It means what we *believe* drives our behavior, both as patients and as providers of care.

If you *believe* that you have no purpose on this planet and that everything is an accident, then you'll likely translate that to your body as well, seeing it as a complex chaos that's impossible to understand and needs help from drugs or surgical procedures. "Germs" are bad and must be eradicated by any means plausible. Conventional medicine is fabulous at determining the bacterial, viral, or fungal entity involved and the best selection of anti-microbials to kill same.

On the other hand, if you *believe* in Intelligent Design or a Creator God, then that means there's an inherent design! Intelligence is at work in the human being and all of creation, whether we recognize or understand that intelligence or not. (Ah, the wonderful mystery!) Even if we don't know why *Streptococcus viridans* exists in our throats or *Helicobacter pylori* in our stomachs or *Clostridium dificile* in our colons, there may be a reason it's beneficial for them to exist where they are—beneficial both for us and the microbes.

This is why some people, particularly since 2020, are frustrated with their doctors and conventional medicine: They are experiencing incongruence between what they believe and what their doctors believe, feeling like doctors are "pushing" them to accept treatments they don't want, while they (the patients) don't have the words to express "why" they don't want said interventions.

Vandana Shiva, a quantum-theory-based physicist, explains it like this:

> *"The way you design the world in your mind is the way you relate to it. When you design it as dead matter just to be exploited, you will exploit it. When you design it without any understanding of limits, you will violate the planetary limits.*
>
> *When you design it with deep recognition of interconnectedness, you will nurture those relationships. And this basic recognition is what I drew from my learnings in quantum theory — that nonlocality, nonseparation, interconnectedness ... is the nature of reality."*

Shiva states that the mechanistic paradigm/worldview is based on the assumptions (See? They're unavoidable!) that we are separate from nature and that nature consists of discrete particles separate from each other, which can only relate through violence, force, and action by contact. This way of viewing the world narrows down to "either/or" (light as a wave OR a particle).

Conversely, the quantum paradigm/worldview is based on the assumptions that there is no separation—everything is, indeed, connected to everything else. In this view, "potential" is a defining quality, and uncertainty rules (German physicist Werner Heisenberg, 1927). In quantum physics, there is no "either/or": light can be a wave AND a particle, which we know to be true. What appears to be different, in this interconnected way of looking at the world, is actually different *expressions* of an interconnected whole.

Belief drives behavior. That's a basic assumption throughout this book.

Personally, I believe in a Creator God and that all humans are made in God's image. I believe that, because of the Creator's wisdom, we have the inherent ability to heal—because we were created for health. We live in a fallen world, so bad things definitely happen. Bones break, harsh words are spoken, the planet is dying from our pollution. We seem to have "forgotten" how to eat real food and drink clean water. Germs overgrow in our systems. However, rather than subduing or eradicating those "germs," I'm interested in *why* they overgrew in the person who's sick with them. If *Streptococcus* lives in our throats but we only get sick with *Strep* when it overgrows, how was the patient living that allowed the germ to overgrow its normal boundaries? And what beneficial aspect might *Strep* in our throats bring to us?

To answer that question from my worldview/medical paradigm, I'd say the pain of overgrown *Streptococcus* in a human throat is the body's inherent wisdom saying, "Hey, there, person of mine. You've been living out of balance lately. You were screaming incessantly at that ball game (trauma), drinking too much alcohol (pH imbalance), and eating too much sugar (immune system suppression). So… here's some pain to jolt you back into balanced living!"

Think about it. Whatever belief system you hold, your physical frame (body) is your closest, long-term friend. It moves you, protects you, and provides your outward identity. Your body remembers everything that ever happened and processes those experiences in the past with information from the present to help inform your next steps into the future.

Your body will—almost literally!—**speak** through physical ailments, emotional upheavals, and the very words that come out of your mouth to give your medical history. If the listening practitioner has the time, training, and a worldview to appreciate your inherent wisdom, the language you choose to tell your story will give that practitioner the information to know exactly where to begin and what to address.

Who's still with me?

Conventional medicine clearly holds the monopoly in medicine, spanning the globe. And it's *fabulous* for emergency care. But applying the short-term "fix" as a long-term plan carries tremendous potential for a negative outcome. That's called "iatrogenesis," which means "harm by medicine" or "harm caused by the physician." This is not medical negligence; rather, it's the right drug or procedure for the right patient, administered the right way by the right provider. You can get medicine at the right time and in the right dosage—yet there's a *wrong* outcome.

The example I gave above happens all the time. A person (let's call him "Bob") is diagnosed with high blood pressure and given a prescription for a beta-blocker. The prescription is written for the correct drug at the correct dose with the correct timing for the correct person, filled correctly by the pharmacist, taken correctly by the patient. Three months later, Bob goes back to the doctor for a follow-up and is given a prescription for a *higher* dose of the same beta-blocker (replacing the original prescription) *plus* a second prescription for another drug to help lower the blood pressure some more.

Wait. What's going on here? Wasn't the first prescription enough? Yes. And no. Hold on, there's more. I'll explain it all.

More months go by, and Bob goes back to the doctor for some blood work. His cholesterol has gone up, so he gets—you guessed it!—refills on the two blood pressure-lowering agents and a brand-new prescription for a cholesterol reducer (a statin). Within a year, Bob is diagnosed with type 2 diabetes.

That, my readers, is iatrogenesis. Bob's initial condition was treated in a way that caused other conditions. By conservative numbers, iatrogenesis is the third leading cause of death in the US, right after cardiovascular disease and cancer. Other numbers suggest iatrogenesis is the *leading* cause of death in the US and has been for several decades.

Wow. I know! Here's what happened to Bob…

Beta-blockers do what their name suggests: they block beta receptors. There are beta receptors in the heart; blocking them brings blood pressure down. But the lungs also have beta receptors; blocking them makes breathing more restricted. And those receptors are also in fat stores; blocking them causes the metabolism of cholesterol to become faulty. Either because of its mechanism of action (a direct effect) or depletion of specific nutrients (an indirect effect), beta-blockers are well-known for causing disruption to both cholesterol and blood glucose regulation. In other words, beta-blockers can CAUSE lipid abnormalities (next diagnosis: dyslipidemia in the form of hypercholesterolemia, hypertriglyceridemia, or hyperlipidemia) and increases in blood glucose (next diagnosis: type 2 diabetes).

The statins—the most commonly used class of cholesterol-reducing medication—are a known cause of type 2 diabetes!

WHAT?

It's true. Pfizer, the maker of statin Lipitor (and many other pharmaceuticals), is embroiled in a class-action lawsuit for pushing patients into type 2 diabetes. (Hey, maybe you qualify! Check here to see: https://usalegal.com/lipitor-class-action-lawsuits/)

Beta-blockers, like any other pharmaceutical, must be given over and over and over again to continue to tell the body what to do. The body, on the other hand, pushes back against the medication. That's called the Law of Dual Effect. The first effect is the drug telling the body what to do; it is temporary. The second effect is the body pushing back against the drug. That effect is lasting. Until the next dose of medication starts the cycle again!

Fun Fact about Fleetwood…

I ride a motorcycle! In the event that I'm sideswiped by a car while on my "beau'iful Bri'ish bike" (read that with an English accent, please), I WANT conventional medical care! I want the heroics that helped make conventional medicine the giant that it is today. As much as I adore vitalistic naturopathic care, having my colleagues rush to my aid with arnica and yarrow aren't going to cut it if my need is for morphine, surgery, and a possible blood transfusion. After conventional medicine saves my life, however, I want my naturopathic friends to restore me to vibrant health!

Statins have their greatest cholesterol-lowering effect with the very first dose. Subsequent dosing never pushes the number any lower than that first dose. Why? Because the body, in its wisdom, begins making extra cholesterol for a darn good reason—cholesterol has an important role in the body. It's the backbone of our sex hormones and it's necessary for cognitive functioning—the rate of dementia has steadily climbed since statins came on the market—and cholesterol helps to line inflamed vessels so they don't rupture. (The current best theory for cholesterol being so high as to be problematic is that it is the body's attempt to address inflammation. The older idea was that it came from eating red meat or eggs or butter.)

Alas, too much of a good thing can become problematic. But lowering cholesterol or high blood pressure or blood glucose without teaching the person how to live differently is, in my opinion, missing the point and putting the patient's life at risk.

Conventional medicine and its doctors bank on the *first* effect—what the drug forces the body to do. Vitalist naturopathic medicine and its doctors bank on the *second* effect—how the body responds to the "medicine" (whether that's an herb, a homeopathic remedy, craniosacral therapy, or a water treatment). We're *wanting* what the body will do in response to the primary effect. Our medicine is often given only once. (Who can make money off *that* model? Not drug manufacturers, for sure.)

Here's an overlooked, unasked question: What might have given Bob high blood pressure in the first place? There's a list of medications for other complaints that can cause blood pressure to rise sufficiently for the diagnosis of hypertension to be given (Appendix A, Table 1). Maybe he was taking acetaminophen for headaches or joint pain. Maybe he was taking gabapentin for nerve pain. Maybe he has an issue with heavy metals that has yet to be discovered, or an underactive thyroid gland. Maybe he's just overweight and stressed out! All of these things and more can cause hypertension.

Recognized Personal Biases, and Noteworthy Beliefs.

According to the Cambridge dictionary, a bias is *the action of supporting or opposing a particular person or thing in an unfair way because of allowing personal opinions to influence judgment.*

That same dictionary defines a belief as *the feeling of being certain that something exists or is true.*

Biases and beliefs are linked. I have a few of each. You might write to inform me of a few other biases after reading this book. That's fine. My biases because of my beliefs include…

- Heroic conventional medicine saves lives. Vitalist naturopathic medicine saves lives, too, and also saves marriages and families and the communities it serves. We're working to save the planet as best we can, despite our small numbers.
- There's a time and a place for nearly every drug currently on the US market. There are a few drugs that I think are particularly frightening because of their *Boxed Warnings* and too few trials, which are often prescribed as if they were benign. This *laissez-faire* attitude puts patients' lives at risk. The first principle of *medicine* (not just vitalist naturopathic medicine) is, "Do No Harm"—do *not* put patients' lives at risk.

Before We Begin...

- Conventional medicine in the US is a broken, corrupt system of disease-management. Again, it's useful in a catastrophic crisis—to put back together a body disrupted by an accident or mishap, for example. But I've met far too many people—from my pharmacy days to my physician days—who have failed with conventional medicine or have been failed by it, at best. At worst, some were actually harmed by conventional medicine.

- Vitalist naturopathic medicine is a far kinder and gentler medicine—a restoration of health-focused medicine. It is an empowering, profound, wholistic approach that includes the direct participation of the patient/client. In fact, without the direct participation of the patient/client, no actual change can occur in the human body. Prescriptions can change the numbers or quiet the symptoms, but what does that do for the patient? In many cases, it sends them right back into the same *lifestyle* that made them sick in the first place!

- Complementary and Alternative Medicine (CAM) should mean treatments that complete something else (complementary) or provide a different option (alternative). Conventional medicine calls anything that is not itself "CAM," but in fact, they don't cooperate with CAM practitioners or consider it an option. "Complementary" means to offset mutual deficiencies and enhance mutual strengths. "Alternative" means offering a choice. Do you see that happening in medicine? Conventional medicine is doing all it can to quash "CAM" and their practitioners, not enlist their cooperation. And while alternative medicine implies choice, many states allow only one choice. In Florida, it's a felony offense to practice CAM if you're *not* also an MD or DO. How "complementary" or "alternative" is that?

- Most people choose one kind of medicine or the other. Some use both simultaneously with good results. I suppose I could offer nutritional advice or supplement recommendations to "complement" the conventional medicine one may choose to take. I could offer therapies to ease suffering that's otherwise being suppressed by medication. But if I believe a particular worldview that is not shared by my client, we'll both start to feel that tension very quickly in our working relationship. In other words, at some point there must be a clear decision or choice of one direction in care or the other. Philosophically, there's a divide.

- Our overall worldviews affect our medical choices. I've been vilified, lied about, shadow-banned and "canceled" by people who disagree with my medical worldview—not so much by people who disagree with my belief in who God is, but by those whose medical paradigm/worldview is at odds with mine. Those who believe that there is a higher power—be it the One I accept as the Most High God, or a different god from a different world religion, or even a personal higher "self"—rarely take issue with me. But those who see the world as inherently chaotic and dangerous seem to view me the same way. Fascinating!

- Every person being given a prescription or procedure ought also to be given the whole story about same. A *Boxed Warning* on a drug is only good if the patient reads it. When the governing bodies determine that no *Boxed Warning* is warranted on an anti-convulsant medication, while knowing a patient's suicidal thoughts and tendencies might dramatically increase when taking the drug, they're removing *informed consent*. (All anti-convulsant medications still list suicidal ideation among their precautions, but the strongest warning—the *Boxed Warning*—was downplayed because of the concern that it would discourage patients from taking their medication.) https://pubmed.ncbi.nlm.nih.gov/20388896/

- Every person ought to be taught how to eat real food, drink clean water, play on a daily basis, get restorative sleep, engage in healthy relationships, and live life on purpose. *These are the determinants of health!* Too few people understand this. Every person ought to have these rights, as well. For all the wealth and resources this country has, the lack of food security and having basic needs met is disturbing.
- People in every community ought to have access to a vitalist naturopathic doctor for education and low-force intervention before rushing to the MD's office for symptom control.
- Adverse Childhood Events are likely the biggest single determining factor for poor health outcomes in adulthood on all levels of existence: physical, emotional, mental, and spiritual.
- Environmental toxins are becoming more of a burden in each successive decade. We're to be stewards of this phenomenal planet, not to strip its resources for personal/corporate gain.
- Humans have much more in common with one another than differences. Yet each person is a unique individual. Therefore, as a vitalist naturopathic doctor, I provide individualized care based on the person's needs, desires and beliefs rather than a prescribed protocol for the masses who experience a similar reaction to their environments.

What's Coming Up In this Book?

CHAPTER ONE: "Diseases of the Drugs" in Hypertension
- The drugs that can cause hypertension—your potential past.
- The secondary diagnoses that taking drugs to manage hypertension can cause—your potential present/future.
- Nutritional deficiencies commonly seen in patients with hypertension and the nutritional deficiencies caused by drugs used to manage hypertension—the next potential diagnoses.
- The other ingredients found in anti-hypertensive drugs
- Appendix A and all the Tables associated with hypertension, plus a Rolling Blood Pressure log to print out

CHAPTER TWO: "Diseases of the Drugs" in Cholesterol Abnormalities (Dyslipidemia)
- The drugs that can cause dyslipidemia—your potential past.
- The secondary diagnoses that taking drugs to manage dyslipidemia can cause—your potential present/future.

Before We Begin...

- Nutritional deficiencies commonly seen in patients with dyslipidemia and the nutritional deficiencies caused by drugs used to manage dyslipidemia—the next potential diagnoses
- The other ingredients found in cholesterol/triglyceride-reducing drugs
- Appendix B and all the Tables associated with dyslipidemia

CHAPTER THREE: "Diseases of the Drugs" in Type 2 Diabetes
- The drugs that can cause type 2 diabetes—your potential past.
- The secondary diagnoses that taking drugs to manage type 2 diabetes can cause—your potential present/future.
- Nutritional deficiencies commonly seen in patients with type 2 diabetes and the nutritional deficiencies caused by drugs used to manage type 2 diabetes—the next potential diagnoses.
- The other ingredients found in drugs used to manage type 2 diabetes
- Appendix C and all the Tables associated with type 2 diabetes plus a Rolling Blood Glucose log to print out

WHEN YOU FLIP THIS BOOK OVER (?!), you'll find:
- Disease Reversal
- How to REVERSE hypertension, cholesterol abnormalities, and type 2 diabetes
- Determining when over-medication is happening, both subjectively and objectively
- Where to find competent de-prescribers
- How to talk to prescribers about de-prescribing the drugs
- Multiple exercises to get all your pieces-parts in alignment
- References and Resources, plus a printable one-page reminder of "Naturopathic Basics"

CHAPTER ONE

"Diseases of the Drugs" in Hypertension

Let's make sure we're all still on the same page, so to speak. *Iatrogenesis* means "medical care which can cause pain, sickness, or death." It comes in different forms and from several different directions. It's been an inherent part of medicine from its very beginning. It can act both directly and indirectly, downstream and sideways, in three different ways: through the drug's own action on its target receptor; through interactions with other drugs, foods, and herbs; and/or through nutritional deficiencies caused by the drug. Yes, there are many places where the *right* medication could go very *wrong*.

To be clear, iatrogenesis isn't exclusive to prescription drugs; it also happens with medical procedures. That's a whole other book that I'll let others write. This book will focus on drug-based iatrogenesis, which I like to call "**D**iseases of the **D**rugs." (Another **F**un **F**act about **F**leetwood: I love alliteration!)

Also, to be clear, iatrogenesis is *not* medical negligence; rather, it's the right drug prescribed at the right time for the right reasons, taken by the right person (like you taking metoprolol, as prescribed by your doctor)—but still, here you are with an ailment you didn't see coming. Or maybe you did see it coming but blamed it on your family's genes. (We'll look at that belief shortly.) *Medical negligence* is a surgeon removing the wrong lung/limb/kidney—or removing the right organ but from the wrong patient—or making the wrong diagnosis, leading to the wrong medication choice. These things do happen!

The various other forms of iatrogenesis include:
- *Indirect* iatrogenesis: health policies themselves that are responsible for illness, death, or disease
- *Structural* iatrogenesis: undermining people's agency and competence to deal with their own diseases
- *Social* iatrogenesis: the medicalization of life
- *Cultural* iatrogenesis: destroying traditional ways of dealing with and making sense of pain, sickness, and death (Iatrogenesis: A review on nature, extent, and distribution of healthcare hazards [nih.gov])

While we're defining terms, let's consider *informed consent,* which means "the process in which a healthcare provider educates a patient about the risks, benefits, and alternatives of a given procedure or intervention. The patient must be competent to make a voluntary decision about whether to undergo the procedure or intervention. An ethical and legal obligation." NIH National Library of Medicine (Shah, Thorton)

The way I see it, the patient gets three choices:

1. Do nothing
2. Accept medical management
3. Choose the hard work of disease reversal

The doctor/practitioner, on the other hand, must provide *informed consent* on *all* of the possible interventions—including disease reversal—and then support the patient's medical choice of doing nothing, accepting medical management, or opting for disease reversal.

Iatrogenesis and informed consent, my friends, are two of the reasons I'm writing this book—to bring you knowledge you didn't have before.

This first half of the book is a "downer," I've been told. It *is* about the "diseases of the drugs"—and that means it's not going to be particularly uplifting.

The second half of the book is the *delightful* portion—all about disease reversal, with de-prescribing built right in. But read this half first, so you'll have the full set of information with which to make a truly informed decision. Choosing to reverse a chronic disease is tough; it typically requires a complete lifestyle overhaul. Because I so want you to choose that option, I strongly encourage you to read all of this information. I'll make it as enjoyable as possible.

Here comes some knowledge, so you can choose how to *live*, lest ye perish prematurely!

The drugs that can cause hypertension—your potential past

Appendix A, Table 1 contains commonly prescribed drugs, over-the-counter agents, and lifestyle choices that can actually cause blood pressure to rise, leading to the diagnosis of hypertension or high blood pressure.

Any asthmatics reading this book? Your **beta-agonist inhalers (short-acting and long-acting), steroids, theophylline, and decongestants** might be the cause of your rising blood pressure.

Informed Consent Withheld?

Recently, a student held me after pharmacology class to ask my opinion on his supervising clinic doctor who had prescribed lisinopril to a woman although she'd already stated more than once that she didn't want a prescription. That doctor did not tell her about the potential of developing a dry cough because of that medication. Nor did he offer her disease reversal. Or any other option. I'll let you guess my opinion on that. So many reasons for me to write these books!

"Diseases of the Drugs" in Hypertension

Have you ever taken medications for **depression, anxiety, or bipolar disease**? The drugs used for these diagnoses, as well as every category of "mood stabilizers" (which, by the way, happen to be anti-seizure medications and anti-psychotic agents, other than lithium) can increase blood pressure to the point of clinical hypertension.

Anyone taking **hormones** for any reason? Please don't think you're "safe" because you're using bio-identical hormone replacement, as these substances can cause blood pressure to rise just like synthetic and animal-derived hormones. *Men, don't skip this paragraph!* Testosterone and methyltestosterone fall into this category, too!

Relatively obvious medications and lifestyle choices that raise blood pressure include: prescriptions for **ADD/ADHD, street drugs** ("uppers" like cocaine and methamphetamine), and **socially acceptable "uppers"**—coffee, black tea, caffeinated sodas and super-caffeinated "energy" drinks.

Less obvious medications and lifestyle choices that also can raise blood pressure include: **over-the-counter decongestants, anti-acne/anti-wrinkle agents** (tretinoin/Retin A), and **pain relievers:** acetaminophen/Tylenol, ibuprofen, naproxen, and their other non-steroidal anti-inflammatory (NSAID) cousins—some of which are still available by prescription only and many of which are "hidden" in cold/allergy and sleep preparations. Eating lunch meats preserved with nitrites and nitrates can raise blood pressure. Smoking cigarettes, being overweight or sedentary, consuming processed foods, and overconsuming alcohol can contribute to high blood pressure.

Anti-Parkinson's drugs, anti-migraine drugs, anti-transplant-rejection drugs, anti-auto-immune drugs, and anti-retrovirals can also raise blood pressure.

Here's the bottom line: your current high blood pressure might have been caused by a medication you took, or continue to take, for other symptoms like congestion or pain, or even by over-consuming caffeine in your morning (or all-day) beverages. If you were or are medicated for diagnoses such as acne, depression, ADD/ADHD, migraine headaches, epilepsy, or asthma (among others), those medications can drive blood pressure high enough to cause your prescribing physician to write the next prescription for hypertension control. If you're taking **steroids** for any reason, your blood pressure can go up. Likewise, hormone therapy—bio-identical or synthetic, for contraception or peri/post-menopause, in women or men—can cause blood pressure elevation high enough to warrant a medication to offset this "side effect" of exogenous (external) hormones.

Yes. It's true. You'll notice I used both past and present tense in the last paragraph. If you *were* taking medications…. even though you might not even be taking them any longer, the increase in blood pressure may have already occurred. Sometimes, when the offending agent is removed, blood pressure comes back down; sometimes it doesn't. Rarely does the prescribing practitioner stop to consider if the last prescription written was, indeed, the cause of this new complaint.

Are you starting to see how very widespread iatrogenesis might be? Wait until you see what the drugs offered to *manage* high blood pressure can cause! Before you start down the path of anti-hypertension

> ### Boxed Warnings
>
> These are the Federal Drug Administration's strongest warnings for prescription drugs. Agents carrying Boxed Warnings do so because they also carry significant risks of serious and/or life-threatening side effects.
>
> *Where are these warnings found?* The bold-type warnings are placed in a prominent, outlined, bolded box on the top of the paperwork folded up like origami and wrapped over the top of the manufacturer's stock bottle, which is then placed inside its own cardboard box.
>
> *So, who gets to see these bolded, boxed warnings?* And therein lies the dilemma, Reader! These warnings are part of the packaging that the patients never get to see.

prescription drug use, please consider correcting the issue—and its associated drug "remedy"—that has *caused* the high blood pressure. ☺

The secondary diagnoses that taking drugs to manage hypertension can cause—your potential present/future.

Appendix A, Table 2 contains the drug classes used to manage hypertension, the nutrients they waste, and the future disease states they can cause. Yes, you read that correctly. *Drugs can cause diseases* from their direct actions on the body, as well as from downstream effects. Think of a line of dominoes falling…

Every manufacturer of every drug in this section states that their medication should be used *in conjunction with lifestyle modifications* such as losing excess weight, regular exercise, limiting salt/alcohol intake, and reducing stress levels.

In this section, we'll focus on the drugs' effects; next, we'll look at the nutritional deficiencies these agents can cause and what the next round of symptoms might look like—symptoms that will likely cause your medical doctor to whip out that ever-ready prescription pad.

If you've been prescribed a **thiazide diuretic** such as hydrochlorothiazide (HCTZ for short), chlorothiazide, indapamide, metolazone or chlorthalidone, "latent diabetes may become manifest." *What?* That means these agents can *cause* type 2 diabetes. Granted, the phrasing used still points to lifestyle choices being the ultimate cause of diabetes, with these pharmaceutical agents merely "uncovering" what was already there. If you're with me again in another book in this series about autoimmune disorders, we'll see a *lot* of "latent" problems that "manifest" after initiation of drug therapy. Thiazide diuretics can also make allergies, asthma, kidney disease, and liver disease *worse*.

Here we'll see an ethnicity difference with pharmaceuticals: Black people respond to thiazide diuretics better than white people do. To be clear, the pharmaceutical manufacturers referencing these study results don't specify what "Black" means. Of African descent? Or greater melanin in the skin producing darker coloration? I'm curious because I have Indian-American friends who are darker in color than my African-American friends. How shall I counsel them? Fortunately, I tend to counsel around disease reversal rather than medication management. Certainly, some prescription options are more appropriate than others for a given individual.

If you've been prescribed a **loop diuretic** such as furosemide, bumetanide, or torsemide, your electrolytes can be thrown so out of balance that you can actually experience "profound diuresis" (bumetanide gets a *Boxed Warning* for this potential), which means you can literally pee yourself into circulatory collapse, throwing clots along the way. This does not happen to everyone, and sometimes the potential risk is clearly outweighed by the potential benefit. My argument is that most people are not given this information, thereby negating the ethic of *informed consent*. Loop diuretics can also worsen kidney function and cause "ototoxicity" (hearing loss, ringing in the ears). Usually, the ototoxicity is reversible when the drug is discontinued, but not always.

Maybe your blood pressure is just a little bit high, or you tend to run low in potassium (maybe because of using another medication in this chapter) so your doctor chose a **potassium-sparing diuretic** like spironolactone, eplerenone, triamterene, or amiloride. These agents should be avoided in patients with Addison's disease, diabetes, severe kidney or liver disease, acidosis, or any urination problems.

As their class name implies, these agents hold potassium in the system. Potassium has a very narrow therapeutic range; anything outside that narrow range—above or below—can cause problems in other organs, most notably the heart. While the loop diuretics have the warning of profound diuresis and loss of potassium (bumetanide), the potassium-sparing agents have a *Boxed Warning* for the potential of dangerously *high* potassium (triamterene).

Alpha receptor blockers (antagonists) and potentiators (agonists) include clonidine, guanfacine (used more for kids with ADD/ADHD than adults with hypertension these days), methyldopa, doxazosin, prazosin, and terazosin. Alpha receptors are part of the adrenergic nervous system. **It is dangerous to stop these medications abruptly.** In my early days as a pharmacist, these agents were initially administered in the doctor's office, as they can cause dramatic drops in blood pressure with the very first dose. Because of the Law of Dual Effect, that first dramatic drop, which can be potentially dangerous for highly-perfused organs like the kidneys, isn't likely to happen with repeated dosing. If the patient handled the first dose well in the doctor's office, he'd be given a prescription for the rest of the month to fill at the pharmacy.

Another class of blood pressure-lowering agents affecting the adrenergic nervous system are **beta-blockers**. Doctors typically start these medications at low doses, then gradually increase the strength over time. Conversely, when it's time to de-prescribe, doctors must very gradually decrease the dosage strength, so as to minimize exacerbating angina and/or causing a heart attack. Beta-blockers include atenolol, propranolol, nadolol, timolol, penbutolol, sotalol, pindolol, labetalol, metoprolol, acebutolol, bisoprolol, esmolol, betaxolol, and carvedilol. Not all of these are used for hypertension; some are used as anti-arrhythmics.

First-generation beta-blockers are non-selective, meaning they'll affect the heart and vascular smooth muscle (good for lowering blood pressure) but also the kidneys, lungs, gastrointestinal tract, uterus, and skeletal muscle. Second-generation beta-blockers are more specific for the beta receptors in the heart. Both generations tend to worsen lung function. That makes sense anatomically and physiologically because the heart and lungs are so intimately connected. When a pharmaceutical drug like a beta-blocker is given to correct a heart issue, that makes breathing more difficult for the asthmatic patient (who likely has a beta-*agonist* on hand as a "rescue inhaler").

All the beta-blockers get the FDA's strongest warning about abrupt discontinuation. One standout in this class is sotalol AF (which stands for "atrial fibrillation" and/or "atrial flutter," additional indications for use of sotalol). Its *Boxed Warning* includes worsening of ventricular tachycardia, atrial fibrillation, and atrial flutter. (*Wait! Sotalol AF can worsen the very thing it's supposed to help? Yes. It can.*)

Beta-blockers tend to be cleared faster in Black people, rendering them likely less useful.

But take heart (pun intended), my friends and family members of color! **Calcium channel blockers** typically work better for Black people. They do carry the risk of gingival hyperplasia (overgrowth of gum tissue in the mouth) and should not be used as a "quick fix" for acutely high blood pressure, nor for the control of "essential hypertension," nor within the first week or so after a heart attack or in a patient likely to have a heart attack in the near future. "Essential hypertension" means no medical cause can be found for the blood pressure being elevated. This diagnosis accounts for 90 to 95 percent of all hypertensive cases. *Wow!*

The **calcium channel blockers** include amlodipine (works more in the legs through vasodilation than in the heart), felodipine, nisoldipine, isradipine, levamlodipine, nifedipine, diltiazem, and verapamil (these last two work more in the heart than in the legs). All require monitoring of potassium levels.

These next two classes of blood pressure-lowering agents are related: **angiotensin converting enzyme (ACE) inhibitors** and **angiotensin receptor blockers (ARBs)**. The ARBs work just upstream from the ACE inhibitors and warrant fewer precautions. They both have the same *Boxed Warning* about fetal and neonatal morbidity and mortality. These agents should not be offered to women of childbearing potential because they can kill the baby, should the patient become pregnant. Both can cause malignancies and kidney failure; both can cause potassium levels to rise. Both are less beneficial in Black patients. ACE inhibitors increase the risk of angioedema (which can be life-threatening) in Black patients. The ACE inhibitors also cause a dry, non-productive cough in about 20 percent of the patient population taking them, making them lousy options for performers and speakers.

ARBs include losartan, olmesartan, valsartan, candesartan, irbesartan, telmisartan and azilsartan kamedoximil. (Wouldn't you love the job of naming new drug entities?)

The ACE inhibitor family includes lisinopril, enalapril, ramipril, benazepril, quinapril, moexipril, fosinopril, captopril, trandolapril, and perindopril.

"Diseases of the Drugs" in Hypertension

Time for Some Self-Assessment

Let's stop here long enough for you to make a list of everything that's "wrong" with you. Really! It might read like this: high blood pressure, ringing in the ear, difficulty falling or staying asleep, weird dreams, cough, decreased sex drive, high cholesterol, pre-diabetes, blood pressure *increases*, concern of auto-immune condition (lupus or even cancer). Have you had a heart attack or stroke since being medicated for high blood pressure? All of the things listed above—and more—can happen from taking anti-hypertensive medications. That's how serious iatrogenesis can be.

Tell me, Reader, what's "wrong" with your health at this point in time?

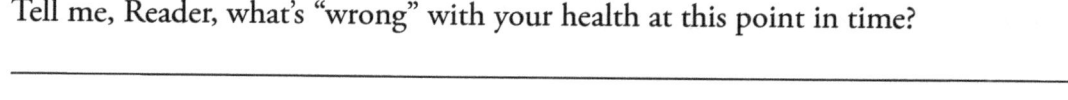

How much of what you just listed may have been caused by your anti-hypertension medication? See why *informed consent* is so important? How much of the above information did your prescriber warn you about? It's rather outrageous, wouldn't you agree? But please don't call your doctor while outraged. When I point out problems, I also offer solutions. Just stay with me, gather more precious knowledge along the way, and I'll give you scripts for speaking with your provider, should you choose to take a different path. In the meantime, **do NOT take yourself off any prescription medications!**

"Knowledge is power." —Sir Francis Bacon.

I mostly agree. I'd suggest this revision:

"Knowledge is power *when put into practical application*." —Dr. Christie Fleetwood

Nutritional Deficiencies Caused by Drugs Used to Manage Hypertension—Those Potential Next Diagnoses

Appendix A, Table 3 contains the disease states that can happen from poor nutrition. Maybe that's what caused the high blood pressure in the first place! Once on medication management, the nutrients that the drugs deplete can then cause additional nutritional deficiencies and subsequent diagnoses of disease. But there's good news! Table 3 also provides the **food sources** of those medication-depleted nutrients.

In the last section, did your list of everything that's wrong with you include any of these problems:

> fatigue, irritability, weakness, muscle tightness/spasms, sugar cravings, poor nail growth, anxiety, painful menstrual cycles, poor concentration, memory lapses, heart skipping beats or racing, abdominal bloating, osteoporosis, hyperactivity, periodontal disease, prostate changes, vision changes, altered taste perception, increased sensitivity to pain, Seasonal Affective Disorder (SAD) or other "negative" mood changes, disordered thinking, anorexia, indigestion, constipation, edema, muscle wasting, nausea, itchy/

dry scalp or skin, sores on mucous membranes (inside nose, mouth), tongue swelling, getting sick frequently, shortness of breath, aching bones/joint, easy bruising, bleeding gums, swollen joints, poor growth, eczema, hot flashes?

Whatever you listed, don't despair! It's daunting and frustrating and maybe a bit infuriating to find out, after-the-fact, that the drugs you've been taking to *help* you have potentially caused suffering. I've witnessed this over and over again. It's become a defining point of my naturopathic practice. I'll share plenty of information to help you get out of the place you now find yourself.

Here are the nutritional deficiencies associated with blood pressure medications and the conditions to which they contribute:

- **Calcium deficiency**: Osteoporosis, osteomalacia, muscle spasms, **hypertension**, periodontal disease, hyperactivity, anxiety, insomnia. Calcium is wasted by loop and thiazide diuretics, the potassium-sparing diuretic triamterene, and the calcium channel blocker amlodipine.
- **Chromium deficiency: Blood sugar irregularities, elevated cholesterol and triglycerides**. Chromium is depleted by beta blockers.
- **Coenzyme Q-10 deficiency**: Fatigue (mentally and physically). CoQ-10 is depleted by thiazide and loop diuretics, as well as by beta blockers.
- **Folate deficiency**: Poor growth, megaloblastic anemia, swollen tongue, GI disturbances. Folate is depleted by loop diuretics and the potassium-sparing diuretic triamterene.
- **Magnesium deficiency**: Fatigue, irritability, weakness, muscle tightness/spasms, menstrual irregularities, **hypertension**, cardiomyopathy, nerve conduction problems, anorexia, insomnia, **sugar cravings**, poor nail growth, anxiety. Thiazide and loop diuretics deplete magnesium.
- **Melatonin deficiency**: Poor sleep, irregular sex hormone production (affecting menstrual cycles, fertility, sexual desire, overall health). Melatonin is a hormone secreted by the pineal gland in response to sunlight. Beta blockers diminish the ability of our pineal glands to produce this hormone.
- **Potassium deficiency**: Fatigue, muscle weakness, mental confusion, irritability, arrhythmias, muscle cramps, abdominal bloating, nerve conduction issues. Potassium is depleted by thiazide and loop diuretics as well as the calcium channel blocker amlodipine.
- **Sodium deficiency**: Altered acid-base balance, altered electrical activity, disrupted water balance, kidney/adrenal dysfunction. Thiazide and loop diuretics deplete sodium, as do ACE inhibitors.
- **Vitamin B1 (Thiamin) deficiency**: Disordered thinking, mental confusion, irritability, anorexia, muscle weakness and tenderness, indigestion, constipation, tachycardia, palpitations, swelling, difficulty walking, muscle wasting. Loop diuretics deplete thiamin.
- **Vitamin B6 (Pyridoxine) deficiency**: Depression, nausea, vomiting, lesions on mucous membranes, seborrheic dermatitis, peripheral neuritis, hearing disorders, irritability, altered mobility and alertness, abnormal movements of body parts, convulsions. Loop diuretics deplete pyridoxine.

- **Vitamin B12 (Cobalamin) deficiency**: Pernicious anemia, fatigue, depression, confusion, memory loss, psychosis, tongue swelling, lack of hydrochloric acid in gut, poor immune system response, spinal degeneration. Loop diuretics deplete cobalamin.
- **Vitamin C deficiency**: Fatigue, weakness, shortness of breath, muscle cramps, aching bones/joint/muscles, anorexia, dry skin, fever, hemorrhage, easy bruising, swollen joints, bleeding gums. Loop diuretics deplete vitamin C.
- **Vitamin D deficiency**: Poor bone health, Seasonal Affective Disorder, increased sensitivity to pain. Thiazide diuretics and the calcium channel blocker amlodipine depletes vitamin D.
- **Vitamin E (mixed tocopherols/tocotrienols) deficiency**: Dry skin, easy bruising, decreased clotting time, eczema, psoriasis, elevated heavy metals, pre-menstrual syndrome (PMS), cystic fibrosis, sickle cell anemia, beta thalassemia, cataracts, fibrocystic disease, enlarged prostate (BPH), poor wound healing, hot flashes, growing pains (including Osgood-Schlatter disease). Loop diuretics deplete vitamin E.
- **Zinc deficiency**: Altered cholesterol synthesis, altered protein synthesis, **altered fat synthesis**, prostate changes, vision changes, **insulin dysregulation**, decreased immune system function, altered taste perception, loss of protection against heavy metal toxicity. Thiazide and loop diuretics, the potassium-sparing diuretic triamterene and ACE inhibitors all waste zinc.

Other Interesting Facts About Hypertension

Vitamin C, calcium, and magnesium are the nutrients that tend to be lacking in most hypertensive patients.

Lead poisoning can be a cause of hypertension, which is one reason why leaded gasoline was banned. It's easy to think about lead poisoning as being a hazard for certain professions, like plumbers, glass manufacturers, printers, plastics or battery manufacturers, and construction workers. But lead can also be found in our drinking water, many canned foods, and old paint.

Another heavy metal that can cause high blood pressure is **cadmium**, also found in drinking water (metal and plastic pipes), fertilizers, cigarette smoke and in the manufacturing of plastics, batteries, paints, textiles and fertilizers.

Hypothyroidism can also be a cause of hypertension.

The Case For Calcium

You don't know what you don't know, right? As a society, we have recently learned a great deal more about nutrition.

Remember when you were drinking milk and eating cheese, listening to the commercials featuring your favorite celebrities with "milk mustaches" waxing eloquently about the benefits of calcium from dairy sources, ending with "Got milk?"

I'll bet you never considered the following:

Cows, goats, sheep; dogs, cats, and kangaroos—all mammals that feed their babies milk—wean their babies from milk at young ages. Except the human mammal. We consume dairy through the lifetime… (wait for it!)… and **it's not even from our own species!** (YUCK.)

Where does the adult cow get her calcium? If she's a CAFO cow (from a Concentrated Animal Feeding Operation), she doesn't! Her dairy products will be fortified with calcium, usually from ground up dead coral or oyster shells. (When was the last time you sat down to a delicious meal of ground up rocks and shells?)

If she's a free-range cow, she gets calcium from her main food source: grass. *So, should we eat grass?* Nope. I've tried it. There's too much cellulose in grass for humans to get the calcium contained therein. We have one stomach; cows have just one stomach, too, but its four separate compartments are designed to allow complete breakdown of their very fibrous diets, including absorption of calcium and other minerals. Great options for single-stomached humans to get bioavailable calcium are turnip greens, torula yeast, lambs quarters (greens), sardines (eat the tiny, soft bones), collard greens, rhubarb, and spinach.

Oh! And did you know (because I just found out) that roughly 65 percent of the human population is lactose intolerant? No kidding! Some nation populations are *100 percent* lactose intolerant! https://worldpopulationreview.com/country-rankings/lactose-intolerance-by-country

And please, *please* do not rush out and buy bags of supplements! You *cannot* cure what ails you with more pills! Our bodies are designed to take in nutrition in the form of food. Choose nutrient-dense foods to consume!

Bear with me as I give you a little bit more knowledge. It's a double-edged sword, I know. This last piece of information is the list of the "other ingredients" in the drugs used to lower blood pressure (at the risk of all listed above).

The Other Ingredients Found in Anti-Hypertensive Drugs

Appendix A, Table 4. This is not an exhaustive list, and not every excipient is wholly evil. Having made capsules and tablets as a pharmacist in a compounding pharmacy, I understand "excipients"—the "other ingredients" that go into a formula for various reasons. An excipient might be added to color or flavor a medication, although neither of those is "necessary" for adults to swallow a pill. Others might be used more for the ease of the machines in rapid manufacturing of large quantities of tablets or capsules at a time. What I've written about below are excipients that, in my professional opinion, are potentially hazardous to human health and I can find no reasonable explanation for their inclusion in medications that are being prescribed for people already struggling with some aspect of their health.

NOTE: Much of this information was taken from the Environmental Working Group's website and Ruth Winter's excellent book, *A Consumer's Dictionary of Food Additives.*

- **Ammonium hydroxide**—A caustic inorganic base, persistent (it'll never decompose) or bioaccumulative (it builds up in the body), moderate to high toxicity concerns. Expected to be toxic or harmful. Prohibited for use in food—yet the *Food and Drug* Administration deems it safe for drugs!

- **Anhydrous lactose**—Generally not a problem, except for all the people who are lactose intolerant.
- **Black iron oxide (exterior shell)**—Persistent, bioaccumulative in wildlife and humans. Limited evidence of respiratory toxicity. Limited/incomplete evidence of cancer.
- **Butyl alcohol/n-butyl alcohol (exterior shell)**—Known human lung and skin toxicant. Expected to be toxic or harmful.
- **Corn/maize starch**—I'm not concerned about "corn" unless it's genetically modified and contaminated with glyphosate, a known toxin to humans. At this point in time, about 94 percent of the corn (and soy) grown in the USA is GMO. https://www.nongmoproject.org/blog/the-gmo-high-risk-list-corn/
- **Crospovidone, polyvinyl-polypyrrolidone (PVP), povidone**—Expected to be toxic or harmful.
- **D&C (Drugs and Cosmetics) Yellow #10**—A synthetic dye produced from petroleum or coal tar. Contamination concerns: zinc, aniline, and cadmium. Possible immune and nervous system effects. Allergenic. Endocrine disruptor.
- **D&C Yellow #10 Lake**—A coal tar- or petroleum-produced pigment adhered to aluminum. High concern for contamination: zinc, aniline, cadmium. Cancer concern. Endocrine disruption.
- **D&C Red #27 Aluminum Lake**—A coal tar- or petroleum-produced pigment adhered to aluminum. Persistent, bioaccumulative. Expected to be toxic or harmful. Endocrine disruption.
- **D&C Red #30 Aluminum Lake**—A coal tar- or petroleum-produced pigment adhered to aluminum. Expected to be toxic/harmful. Endocrine disruption.
- **D&C Red #28**—A synthetic dye made from petroleum or coal tar. Persistent, bioaccumulative. Moderate to high toxicity concerns. Expected to be toxic or harmful. Endocrine disruption.
- **D&C Red #33**—Contamination concerns: biphenyl-2-ylamine.
- **Ethyl cellulose**—Ethyl ether of cellulose. Expected to be toxic or harmful to humans. Prohibited for use in food.
- **Ethyl acrylate copolymer**—Ethyl acrylate is a reactive monomer that is highly irritating to the eyes, skin, and mucous membranes. Carcinogenic.
- **FD&C (Food, Drug, and Cosmetics) Blue #1**—Contamination concerns: aniline, cadmium. Neurotoxin. Endocrine disruptor. Moderate cancer concern. Produced from petroleum. Textile dye, wood stain, colorant. Triarylmethane dye.
- **FD&C Blue #1 Aluminum Lake**—A typically synthetically produced dye from petroleum or coal tar. Precipitated to aluminum. Contamination concerns: aniline, cadmium. Banned or found unsafe in cosmetics. Persistent or bioaccumulative with moderate to high toxicity

concerns. Classified as medium human health priority. Limited evidence of carcinogenicity. Used in food or as additive with limited to no toxicity information. Concern of neurotoxicity at any dose. Associated with endocrine disruption.

- **FD&C Red #3**—Banned in cosmetics. Persistent or bioaccumulation concerns.
- **FD&C #40**—A synthetic dye made from petroleum. Contamination concerns: mercury, aniline, cadmium, and 6-methoxy-M-toluidine. Moderate evidence for human allergen or toxicant. Mutation evidence in mammals. Associated with endocrine disruption.
- **FD&C Red #40 Aluminum Lake**—A coal tar- or petroleum-produced pigment adhered to aluminum; concern with contaminants: mercury, 6-methoxy-m-toluidine, aniline, and cadmium. Possible human toxicant or allergen; possible neurotoxin; mutation results on mammalian cells; persistent and bioaccumulative in wildlife; endocrine disruptor.
- **FD&C Yellow #6 Aluminum Lake**—A petroleum or coal tar derivative precipitated to metal salt, typically aluminum (or calcium, barium, or other). Contamination concern with cadmium. Moderate evidence of human toxicant or allergen. Possible neurotoxin and reproductive/developmental harm. Associated with endocrine disruption.
- **Glyceryl triacetate, triacetin**—Expected to be toxic or harmful.
- **Hydrogenated vegetable oil**—A *trans fat*, usually made from soybeans. About 94 percent of soybeans grown in US are GMO. Concern for glyphosate contamination. Contains MSG.
- **Isopropyl alcohol (exterior shell)**—First commercial synthetic alcohol. Reaction of propylene (petroleum byproduct) with sulfuric acid, then hydrolysis. The US government has regulations in place for the amount of isopropyl alcohol allowed in foods.
- **Light mineral oil**—A byproduct of the petroleum industry. Eye irritant. Causes birth defects and cancer by inhalation. Strong evidence of respiratory toxicant or allergen. Expected to be toxic or harmful. (Pills aren't rubbed in the eye nor are they inhaled. This is also used medically as a liquid to be ingested for constipation, yet it's expected to be toxic or harmful. Why is it part of pharmaceutical manufacturing?)

Mag Stearate

Used in fast-manufacturing of pharmaceuticals AND nutraceuticals, this fat is a lubricating agent, lining the interior tubing for capsules and their contents. Think about that, Reader. If magnesium stearate is lining the tubing where the herbs or vitamins or active medicinal agents are being sent whizzing down those tubes, won't they then be coated with this fat? In the presence of oxygen, fats become rancid. Our cells require fat and will use whatever fats we give them, incorporating the fats right into the cell membranes.

Rancid, inappropriate fats in human cell membranes are a fast-track to cell death.

- **Magnesium stearate**—This ingredient has become a deal-breaker for me when selecting supplements for my clients. It gets its own side-bar comment.
- **Methacrylic acid**—Use is restricted in Canadian cosmetics. Allowed workplace exposures restricted to low doses. Occupational hazards related to handling. Toxic or harmful.
- **Methyl paraben**—Parabens mimic estrogen. Endocrine disruption. Interferes with gene expression.
- **Methylene chloride/dichloromethane**—A known human respiratory toxicant. Limited evidence of gastric or liver toxicity. Banned or found unsafe for use in cosmetics. Possible human carcinogen. Persistent or bioaccumulative in wildlife. Limited evidence of reproductive toxicity.
- **Potassium hydroxide (exterior shell)**—Classified as toxic or harmful. Wildlife and environmental toxicity concern.
- **Propylene glycol (trimethyl glycol, methyl ethyl glycol, dihydroxypropane, propanediol) (external shell)**—A skin irritant; penetration enhancer. Expected to be toxic or harmful. Various grades used in foods, engine coolants, airplane de-icing, antifreeze, enamels, paints. About 45 percent eliminated via kidneys; the rest is turned into lactic acid. Potential interaction with metformin and lactic acid toxicity. (https://www.webmd.com/diet/what-to-know-about-propylene-glycol-in-foods)
- **Propyl paraben**—Parabens mimic estrogen. Strong evidence of endocrine disruption. Significant wildlife and environmental disruption. Strong evidence of human immune toxicant or allergen. Possible human reproductive or developmental toxin.
- **Polyethylene glycol**—A petroleum derivative. Growing concern of anaphylaxis. (https://pubmed.ncbi.nlm.nih.gov/33011299/)
- **Polysorbate and Polysorbate 80/Sorbitan**—Contamination concerns: ethylene dioxide, a known human carcinogen. Unsafe for use in cosmetics, known respiratory toxicant, limited evidence of kidney toxicity, eye/lung/skin irritant, strong evidence of human immune toxicant; not expected to be bioaccumulative or environmental toxin. **Unacceptable** per EWG, 1,4-dioxane (synthetic industrial material, completely miscible in water, unstable at higher temperatures/pressure, explosive with prolonged exposure to light/air, resistant to biodegradation, likely to be carcinogenic, upper respiratory, kidney and liver damage). https://www.epa.gov/sites/default/files/2014-03/documents/ffrro_factsheet_contaminant_14-dioxane_january2014_final.pdf)
- **Saccharin sodium**—Artificial sweetener. Used in food or as additive with limited or no toxicity information available. Limited or incomplete evidence of cancer. Controversial over the years.
- **SD-45 alcohol (external shell)**—A specially denatured alcohol. Grain-derived, considered broadly toxic. Penetration enhancer. Persistent, bioaccumulative in wildlife. Used in food or as additive with little to no toxicity information available. Limited evidence of sense organ, gastrointestinal, or liver toxicity. Limited evidence of cancer. Occupational hazards related to handling. Unknown risk to nervous system.

- **Shellac (external shell)**—A resin secreted by the lac bug in Thailand and India. Used as colorant, food glaze, wood finish. Natural glue.
- **Sodium lauryl sulfate**—A topical irritant. Expected to be toxic or harmful. Suspected to be an environmental toxin.
- **Sodium starch glycolate**— A sodium salt of carboxymethyl ether from rice, potato, wheat, or corn. Medium human health priority.
- **Sodium starch glycolate type-A**— Something new on the market approved by the WHO in 2020. May be sourced from corn, potato, or an "unspecified ingredient". https://precision.fda.gov/ginas/app/ui/substanes/H8AV0SQX4D
- **Sodium hydroxide**—Highly caustic and reactive inorganic base known as "caustic soda." Expected to be toxic or harmful. Medium human health priority. Occupational hazards related to handling.
- **Sodium stearyl fumarate**—Causes skin irritation. Causes serious eye irritation. (PubChem)
- **Strong ammonia solution (external shell)**—Amidase inhibitor and neurotoxin. Manufactured and produced naturally by bacterial processes and breakdown of organic matter.
- **Talc—native/natural**—Sometimes contains aluminum silicate. Can be contaminated with asbestos. Asbestos-free, cosmetic-grade talc is a form of magnesium silicate shown to be toxic and carcinogenic.
- **Titanium dioxide**—A white pigment from minerals. Possible human carcinogen. Expected to be toxic or harmful.
- **Zinc stearate**—Zinc salt of stearic acid. Persistent or bioaccumulative and moderate to high toxicity concerns. Persistent, bioaccumulative in wildlife. Expected to be toxic or harmful. Suspected to be environmental toxin.

If the prescription drugs worked with one pill taken, no worries. But when the pill is taken daily and even multiple times a day, over the long-haul of chronic disease management, a lot of toxic matter is ingested, too.

Nope, folks—you can't get health from a pill. You have never been deficient in lisinopril, HCTZ, nor any other pharmaceutical ingredient.

CHAPTER TWO

"Diseases of the Drugs" in Cholesterol Abnormalities (Dyslipidemia)

The drugs that can cause dyslipidemia—Your potential past

Welcome to Chapter Two! Did you read the introduction on "Assumptions?" If not, please take a moment to do so now. If you don't have hypertension, I'll not complain about you skipping that information. I do supply the definitions of *Iatrogenesis* and *informed consent* in Chapter One, so please ensure you've digested that information before returning here.

No matter how irritated you get over what you're about to read, **do *not* take yourself off your cholesterol-reducing prescription medication! First**, you must be given *informed consent* so that you can decide on your medical choice: to do nothing about your cholesterol problems, to accept medical management for your cholesterol problems, or to opt for disease reversal. (These options were discussed in Chapter One.) Disease reversal is outlined in the second half of this book.

Cholesterol. Poor cholesterol! Cholesterol has gotten such a bad rap over the years. So have the foods that were high in cholesterol. If you've lived as long as I have, you'll remember the time when the public was told not to eat eggs (1970s) because of cholesterol—then it became okay to eat eggs, but not butter. In the 1980s, the culprit was mayonnaise (perhaps still the egg), then it was full-fat dairy products, ushering in fat-free products. Somewhere along the way, red meat was shunned for its cholesterol content.

Where does cholesterol come from? Cholesterol is made in our own brilliant bodies! The liver produces about 80 percent of the cholesterol the body requires, leaving the other 20 percent to come from our food choices.

Cholesterol is absolutely necessary for our brains to function and our sex hormones to be produced. I find it interesting how the numbers have shifted over time, mostly because the makers of drugs that can lower cholesterol have driven that trend. Back in the 1980s-90s, total cholesterol wasn't deemed "high" (requiring medical intervention in the form of prescription medication) until it was over 300. During my years as a pharmacist, I saw that number drop down to 220; now it's 200! In the meantime, while we've been steadily dropping cholesterol levels, have heart attacks or strokes diminished? No. Has dementia skyrocketed? Yes! How about fertility issues? Yes, also on the rise. Libido? Tanking.

Bottom line: We need cholesterol to think and make our sex hormones. We overproduce cholesterol when our vessels become inflamed from things like eating inflammatory foods, which are not the same as cholesterol-containing foods, but can vary from person to person— "one man's meat is another man's poison." (--Titus Lucretius Carus, probably.) We also overproduce cholesterol when we live in "inflammatory conditions" that include stress, frustrating relationships, and irritating jobs. Change the way you live, and you'll change the quality and quantity of cholesterol your body produces.

Appendix B, Table 1. These medications—which you might be taking for a number of ailments—can also affect how your body handles cholesterol. The medications include treatments for fluid accumulation, high blood pressure, heart failure, migraine prevention, angina, schizophrenia, depression, bipolar disorder (I or II), seizures/epilepsy, Tourette's disorder, any autoimmune condition including cancer, organ transplant, contraception, heavy menstrual bleeding, endometriosis, sleep issues, anxiety, peri/post-menopausal symptoms, painful intercourse, gender dysphoria, acne, wrinkles, high cholesterol (!), AIDS/HIV, primary hypogonadism, or osteoporosis.

I may have missed a few.

These medications—including the bile acid sequestrants used for *lowering* total cholesterol—can cause your lipid panel to be all kinds of wonky. (I vote that "wonky" be included in the medical dictionary with the definition: "out of whack; too high, too low, or a combination of each; unnaturally unhealthy.") The bile acid sequestrants *raise* triglycerides. The others *raise* total cholesterol or LDL and/or lower HDL and/or raise triglycerides. The medical condition of having abnormal lipid components is called "dyslipidemia."

The Appendix includes a table of the drugs that can cause dyslipidemia, and they fall into these pharmaceutical classes:

Loop and thiazide diuretics used for edema and hypertension.

Beta-blockers used for hypertension, heart failure, migraine prevention, and angina.

Lithium used for mania. That could be mania alone, mania as part of bipolar disorders 1 or 2, or mania associated with psychosis. It's also sometimes used as a "mood stabilizer" in depression. (*Huh?* I know, Reader; that's a separate book.)

Steroids used for inflammation anywhere in the body.

Hormones for men and women—bio-identical as well as synthetic or horse-derived. Yes, this includes hormonal contraceptives.

Anti-depressants, regardless of why they're prescribed.

Retinoids for acne and wrinkles, also used to treat plaque psoriasis and certain cancers.

Anti-retrovirals used to manage HIV/AIDS.

Monoclonal antibodies or "biologics" used to treat autoimmune disorders, certain cancers, and now osteoporosis and skin rashes.

Bottom line: Before you go down the road of medical management for your dyslipidemia, remember Bob and his hypertension, and consider reversing the issue that got you on the medication above that gave you dyslipidemia in the first place.

Costs to Consider in Medical Management

Let's talk about the money side of medical management. There's the obvious financial cost of the disease and the prescriptions to manage the disease. There's also the financial cost of going back and forth to doctors' offices and pharmacies—even if you're only paying "co-payments." The time involved and energy spent on these pieces of ongoing medical management come with a cost. They can include the cost of being overlooked for a promotion because of missing time from work due to illness and doctor appointments. There's also missed time with family and friends due to illness, appointments, and side effects of the medications being taken. Anyone dosed to bowel-tolerance on metformin knows this.

What do you get in exchange for this cost? Medical management doesn't stop the disease process—this will become more obvious in the type 2 diabetes chapter. Even with the very best management, these conditions can shave years off the patient's expected lifespan, compared to a healthy counterpart. And all those cases where iatrogenesis shows up cost people their personal power and autonomy.

Many people choose medical management; that's fine. My contention is, were they given the **choice** of disease reversal? Did they receive *informed consent*?

Why would people choose to be medically managed once they know disease reversal is an option?

That comes down to what we believe—because belief drives behavior. The sheer effort that is required by those who pursue the disease reversal route can be a factor. Medical management requires little from the patient being managed; he can keep living the way that got him sick in the first place by simply taking pills or shots daily to keep the symptoms "manageable" and the lab values down. But that patient pays the costs listed above.

SPOILER ALERT! The concepts I'll reveal to you in the flip-side of this book are straightforward and simple. Simple, I tell you! However, *simple* does not equal *easy*. Nope. A fitting analogy would be Robert Frost's poem, "The Road Not Taken." Once you choose to say "yes" to disease reversal, all opposing options receive your "no."

The path to vibrant health requires active participation!

Disease reversal is a whole other way of looking at *life*. It's about *health*—and also freedom, autonomy, and wholeness. It's about living on *purpose*, with congruence, and authenticity! And it's about personal responsibility, accountability, and mindfully choosing to live out what we say we believe.

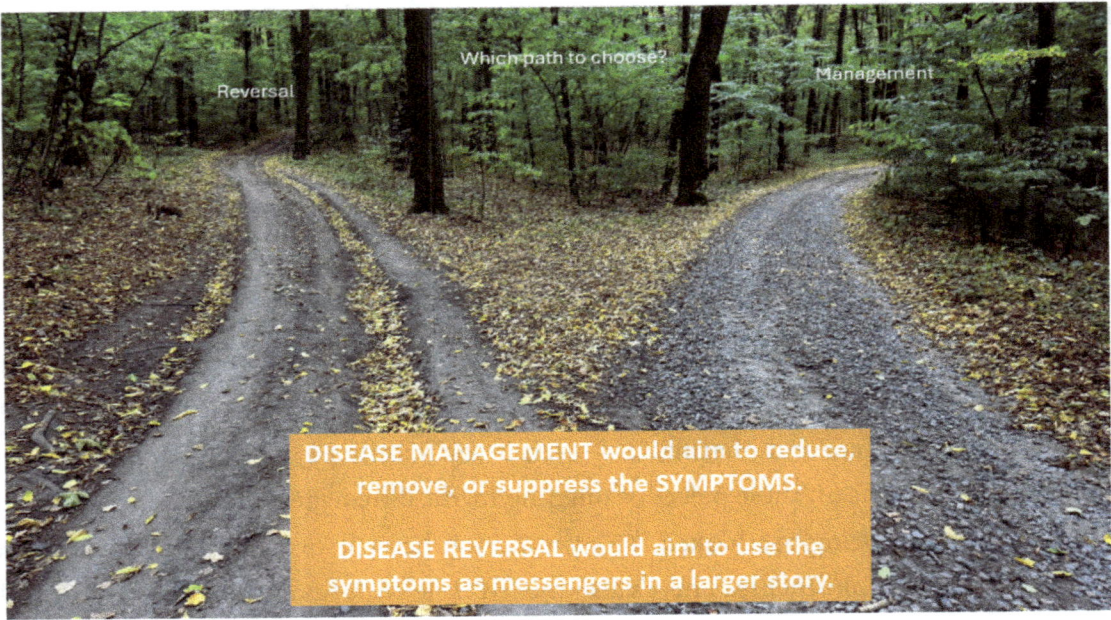

There's that "belief" piece again!

Remember the medical paradigms we looked at in the beginning of this book? If you skipped that part, please go back and read the "introduction," because it's super important in putting all these pieces together. As psychiatrist Iain McGilchrist stated, "The model we choose to use to understand something determines what we find."

For the practitioner, medical management is easier option. Honestly, it's the only option for most physicians, as this is the current paradigm in medicine. Therefore, insurance, education, and workflow—as well as payment structures and research—are all geared for medical management. From the patient's perspective, the doctor needs to determine the correct diagnosis and then choose from the available matching protocols of procedure or prescription. Then the patient just does what he's told.

Disease reversal requires the practitioner to *know more*, including:
- The patient's story, in her own words—the relationships, traumas, and where she was displaced from her own projected trajectory
- The medical history—when he got sick, what else was going on at that time, what diagnoses were made along the way
- The medication history—which drug was selected when and prescribed for what at which dose, and what changes were made to dosing or class over time, and also:
  o what the half-life of each drug is
  o all the iatrogenic possibilities that I'm outlining in this book.

Who's got time for all that in a seven-minute visit? Maybe the time factor influenced the current paradigm, or vice versa. Medical management can be a lucrative business! Who prospers with disease reversal? I'll tell you who prospers, Reader: the patient, his family, his workplace, and his community. But for the past forty, sixty, or eighty years, that has not been the goal in medicine.

From the patient's perspective, in disease reversal, *she's* the one who's got to put all the knowledge into practical application. *She* has to make different decisions to turn her life around for health. *He* has to say "no" to sleeping in and "yes" to going to the gym. The *patient* takes on ultimate responsibility for his/her individual health. The doctor is merely a hired professional to provide direction and counsel. That's a radically different way of practicing medicine!

The Secondary Diagnoses That Taking Drugs To Manage Dyslipidemia Can Cause—Your Potential Present/Future

For those choosing medical management for dyslipidemia, **Appendix B, Table 2** lists the warnings as well as nutrients wasted and the average change in various aspects of the lipid panel afforded by each class. These are even more costs to count!

You'll note that the **bile acid sequestrants**—cholestyramine, colestipol, colesevelam—can increase triglycerides and cause acute pancreatitis. They lower LDL an average of 15 to 30 percent. They can also *cause* constipation (all), GI obstruction (colesevelam, colestipol), chest pain (colestipol) and cancer (colestipol, cholestyramine).

The class of drugs called **fibrates** have really dropped in favor over the years, but they caused their own problems, including decreases in protective HDL while potentially causing liver toxicity, muscle destruction, gall stones, pancreatitis, changes in the health and quality of the blood (bad; very bad), and promote clotting (myocardial infarction (MI), stroke, deep vein thrombosis (DVT), and pulmonary embolism (PE)). They also raise homocysteine, an independent risk factor for many adverse outcomes.

Ezetimibe is in a class all by itself as an **absorption inhibitor**. Interestingly enough, it can cause upper respiratory tract infections, hepatitis, pancreatitis, cholecystitis (gallbladder swelling) and cholelithiasis (gallstones). All the *-itis* endings mean "inflammation." Inflammation is currently considered the root cause of cholesterol being over-produced in the body as a protective measure—an internal band-aid, so to speak—which lines inflamed blood vessels to keep them from rupturing. Alas, too much of a good thing—cholesterol over-lining an inflamed vessel to the point of blocking blood flow—can precipitate a heart attack or stroke. **Ezetimibe** is a drug designed to decrease the amount of cholesterol circulating in the blood stream (looking for places in inflamed vessels) while *increasing inflammation* in the liver, pancreas, and gall bladder. Ezetimibe does tend to decrease total cholesterol on average by 12 points, LDL by 18 points, apolipoprotein B by 16 points, and triglycerides by 8 points, and it can raise HDL by 1 point on average.

The **statins**! These are, far and away, the most commonly prescribed cholesterol-reducers on the market today. The biggest reduction ever seen by these agents happens with the very first dose. That's because of the Law of Dual Effect (which you read about earlier.) This class of agents is absolutely contraindicated in pregnancy due to birth defects and/or death to the developing baby. Remember, cholesterol is necessary for the production of all sex hormones, including those responsible for healthy pregnancy. Statins can also cause painful muscles, destruction of muscles, and immune-driven muscle cell death. *(Yikes!)* It's also implicated in liver dysfunction, endocrine dysfunction, and central nervous system toxicity.

When it comes to altering the lipid panel numbers, statins tend to have the better results compared to the other agents we've already considered, lowering all the "bad" players and raising HDL (rosuvastatin probably "wins" in this family).

There are newer pharmaceuticals on the market now for lowering cholesterol: **monoclonal antibodies (PESK9 inhibitors)** that can cause immune system dysfunction (systemic illness that often goes unnoticed until it's too late to treat). Their number-changing effectiveness exceeds even the statins, so they're gaining popularity. Monoclonal antibodies are used in autoimmune disorders including cancer and have significant warnings and precautions associated with them. The manufacturing process for these agents is quite different from other pharmaceuticals, as they are grown on other critters' pieces and parts. These will be covered extensively in a future book focusing on autoimmunity.

Bempedoic acid is the only agent in the **miscellaneous antihyperlipidemic** category. Notably, it can cause gout and tendon rupture. It's often prescribed as an add-on with a maxed-out statin dose.

Certainly, there are combination products (statin + absorption inhibitor, statin + calcium channel blocker!) and patients taking more than one prescription for cholesterol reduction. What does that tell you? It tells me that taking pills does not change the progression of disease! Every one of these manufacturers states—just as we saw with anti-hypertensive agents and what we will see with anti-diabetic agents—that their products are to be used "adjunct to diet changes." Yet who teaches the patient what changes to make? Not even the "experts" can agree on the nutrition component of dyslipidemia!

Nutritional Deficiencies Caused By Drugs Used To Manage Dyslipidemia

Bile acid sequestrants deplete fat-soluble vitamins (A, D, E, K), omega-3 fatty acids, beta-carotenes, calcium, folate, iron, zinc, vitamins B2, B3, and B12.

That's a lot of wasted nutrition for one drug class! What might the different deficiencies look like?

Let's combine **beta-carotenes with vitamin A**, since they're closely related. A deficiency of these agents could look like vision loss/night blindness, dry eyes, macular

---

Nutrients

Books have been written on differences between the nutrients we get from quality foods vs the nutrients synthesized in laboratories from petroleum industry waste products. Single entity nutrients simply don't exist in nature: "vitamin E" isn't dl-alpha tocopherol succinate; rather, it's d-alpha-, d-beta-, d-delta-, d-gamma- tocopherol with d-alpha-, d-beta-, d-delta-, d-gamma-tocotrienol. Likewise, B vitamins never walk into your blood stream alone; they always come in as a grouping of B vitamins.

degeneration; respiratory infections, follicular hyperkeratosis ("sandpaper skin"), reduced immunity, diarrhea, loss of tooth enamel, loss of bone mass, loss of taste and smell.

Insufficient **vitamin D** can look like malformation or skeletal demineralization of bones. Increased sensitivity to pain. Seasonal Affective Disorder (SAD).

When there's not enough **vitamin E** in your body, you might experience dry skin, easy bruising, decreased clotting (increased bleeding), eczema, psoriasis, elevated heavy metals (due to lack of protection from exposure), PMS, cystic fibrosis, sickle cell anemia, beta thalassemia, cataracts, fibrocystic disease, BPH, poor wound healing, hot flashes, growing pains, or Osgood-Schlatter disease.

Wait a minute! Cystic fibrosis, sickle cell anemia, beta thalassemia? Aren't those inherited genetic traits?

Yes, they are inherited! However, genes cannot code for disease; they make proteins the best they can with the building blocks on hand. If additional nutrients are added—for example, if your lifestyle turns aside from what you were taught to eat in your parents' lifestyle—you might encourage or discourage these diseases from emerging, even after the proteins are made initially. Our brilliantly designed bodies are constantly undergoing renovation, which means inherited conditions can be significantly diminished. If parents were eating a nutritionally dense diet prior to conception, and if the mother's diet remained exceptionally nutritious during the first trimester, 98 percent of these "inherited diseases" would be eradicated.

Vitamin K is necessary for healthy clotting. Low levels of vitamin K can cause hemorrhagic disease of the newborn, spontaneous nosebleeds in children, and osteoporosis.

Omega-3 fatty acids assist in healthy clotting, counterbalancing vitamin K in some ways. Without omega-3 fatty acids, there can be increased clotting, increased inflammation, increased cell permeability, increased triglycerides, and decreased HDL—a "direct 'hit' to the cholesterol dilemma!

Lack of sufficient **calcium** can cause osteoporosis, osteomalacia, muscle spasms/tetany, hypertension, periodontal disease, hyperactivity, anxiety, and insomnia.

A **folate** insufficiency can look like poor growth, megaloblastic anemia, glossitis, and digestive tract disturbances. By the way, folate and folic acid are not the same. Folic acid is man-made and lacks methyl groups; folate is inherent in natural foods and contains all the methyl groups necessary. If you've been told you have an MTHFR mutation, please know that you aren't defective—the stripped-out food you've been consuming is what's defective!

Too little **iron** can cause anemia, glossitis, nail spooning, increased susceptibility to infection, brittle nails, canker sores, hair loss, decreased endurance, and impaired mental ability.

Organic and Regenerative

"Organically-grown" tells us what's **not** in the *produce*: genetically-modified organisms, glyphosate (Roundup is the brand name), other chemical herbicides, insecticides, fungicides, etc.

"Regeneratively-farmed" tells us what *is* in the *soil*: a more diversified ecosystem with greater nutritional density!

Zinc deficiency can cause altered synthesis of cholesterol, protein, and fats and dysregulation of release of vitamin A from liver. Cell growth (epithelial tissue) can be adversely affected, and patients can experience prostate changes, vision changes, insulin dysregulation, immune system lessened, altered taste perception, and loss of protection against heavy metal toxicity.

Without sufficient **B2/riboflavin**—and this typically occurs in concert with other B vitamin deficiencies—patients can develop cheilosis (also known as "angular cheilitis"—sores and cracks in the corners of the mouth), glossitis, dry/scaly skin, itchy eyes, and light sensitivity.

B3/niacin deficiency is classified by its "four Ds": dermatitis (exacerbated by sun exposure), diarrhea, dementia, and death! This deficiency tends to be progressive.

Last but not least, a **B12/cobalamin** deficiency can cause pernicious anemia, progressive peripheral neuropathy with pronounced anemia, fatigue, depression, confusion, memory loss, psychosis, glossitis, and achlorhydria—insufficient acid in the stomach to break down and subsequently absorb nutrition properly, a double whammy! It can also cause impaired lymphocyte response, decreased phagocyte and PMN response, spinal degeneration, and macrocytic cells.

Whew! That was a lot!

It's daunting. Here are the nutritional deficiencies caused by the rest of the cholesterol-reducers:

The **fibrates** aren't quite as problematic as the bile acid sequestrants in causing nutritional deficiencies. Still, they waste vitamin E, zinc, and probably copper and coenzyme Q-10, and they raise homocysteine, an independent risk marker for many diseases. To offset the homocysteine hike, it's worth eating foods rich in B12, B6, and folate. Honestly, if you eat foods rich in nutrition—regeneratively farmed, nutritionally dense foods with a focus on plants—you won't have "need" of a fibrate!

All the nutrients wasted by fibrates except copper, coQ-10 and vitamin B6 are listed above with the bile acid sequestrants (and in **Appendix B, Table 3**). The remaining three are listed here:

A **copper** deficiency can cause red blood cells to break down, anemia, neutropenia, degeneration of vasculature, skin depigmentation, kinky hair, hypotonia, and hypothermia. Copper is essential for moving iron from the liver.

Insufficient **coenzyme Q-10** causes fatigue and diminished energy—both inside the cell and how the individual feels—thereby creating cellular damage.

Lacking **vitamin B6** can cause depression, nausea, vomiting, mucous membrane lesions, seborrheic dermatitis, and peripheral neuritis. It can cause ataxia (clumsy movement), hyperacusis (increased sensitivity to sound), hyperirritability, altered mobility and alertness, abnormal head movements, and seizures.

The **statins** waste coenzyme Q-10 (above, under Fibrates). You might say, *Just that one thing? That's not so bad!* Do you remember seventh-grade Science class, drawing and naming the structures inside a cell? How about the organelle called the mitochondria, the "powerhouse" of the cell where energy is made by turning ADP into ATP? The electron transport chain that makes energy manufacturing possible is powered by coenzyme Q-10. Wasting this one thing ends up being a pretty big deal!

"Diseases of the Drugs" in Cholesterol Abnormalities (Dyslipidemia)

Atorvastatin is the best-selling drug of all time, and it also has a class-action lawsuit against it for pushing people into type 2 diabetes.

The other cholesterol-reducers might also have a nutrient "cost," but none have been discovered as of yet.

Zinc and vitamin D are the nutrients most commonly noted as being deficient in patients with dyslipidemia.

The Other Ingredients Found In Cholesterol/Triglyceride-Reducing Drugs

What would you say to your prescribing physician if she told you that your injectable cholesterol-reducing drug alirocumab/Praluent contained 100 mg of sugar? Or the powdered option of cholestyramine/Questran had more than 3.5 grams of sugar in it? The really ironic thing here is, I bet your prescriber doesn't even know these facts.

But wait! There's more. And it gets worse…

> **Butylated hydroxyanisole (BHA)** is a petroleum-derived preservative banned in Japan for suspected carcinogenic properties.
>
> **Cellacefate** is a polymer phthalate—a concerning and controversial plastic.

Both of these are found in various lipid-lowering prescription drugs.

Some fillers may not be so bad in and of themselves, but there are contamination concerns:

> **Copovidone**: Contamination concerns: vinyl acetate, 1-vinyl-2-pyrrolidone.
>
> **Polysorbate 80**: Contamination concerns: ethylene dioxide (a known human carcinogen, unsafe for use in cosmetics, known respiratory toxicant, limited evidence of kidney toxicity, eye/lung/skin irritant, and strong evidence of human immune toxicant); 1,4-dioxane (a synthetic industrial material, completely miscible in water, unstable at higher temperatures/pressure, explosive with prolonged exposure to light/air, resistant to biodegradation, likely to be carcinogenic, and can cause upper respiratory, kidney and liver damage.)

And these fillers are "expected to be toxic or harmful": crospovidone, sodium lauryl sulphate, triacetin, ammonium hydroxide, potassium hydroxide, and propylene glycol.

Why? Why are ingredients like this in medicine? I share your sentiment, Reader. Check the Table to see what's in **your** cholesterol-reducer. A cry of outrage may be warranted.

Time for a break. Get up, walk around, drink water, maybe enjoy a healthy snack. Read the label, if it's wrapped, to ensure you're eating real food as opposed to food-flavored chemicals. Other options are listed next. Maybe take the dog to the park. I'll see you back here for type 2 diabetes…

Healthy Snack Options

- **Sliced fruits** (apples, pears, bananas) with seed/nut butters (sunflower, pumpkin, peanut, almond, cashew, and/or macadamia). Add raisins for additional flavor, color, and fun in creating various shapes to eat!
- **Vegetable sticks** (carrots, celery, broccoli, cauliflower, cucumbers) with hummus, baba ganouj, or any flavorful (chemical free!) dip.
- **Trail mix**: dark chocolate chips added to a blend of seeds, nuts, and assorted dried fruits.
- **Popcorn** (NOT microwaved!) with salt, grated cheese, and/or nutritional yeast sprinkled on top.
- **Cheese and crackers**. At our house, we use goat, sheep, and water buffalo-milk cheeses and yogurts because they have undergone less processing and "tampering" than cow dairy products. And there's nothing better than water buffalo (bufala) milk mozzarella!
- **Caprese salad**: Slice that wonderful water buffalo-milk mozzarella cheese, place it on a slice of tomato, top it off with a fresh basil leaf, then drizzle a bit of balsamic vinegar over it. Yummy!
- **Seasonal "fun" fruits** like pomelo, pomegranate seeds, starfruit, blood oranges, horned melons, lychees.
- **Baked root vegetables**, such as sweet potatoes, parsnips, carrots, and beets: slice thinly, or cut into sticks; brush with olive oil; bake in the oven until nearly crispy.

NOTE: If you're allergic to nuts or anything else listed above, please don't eat it!

CHAPTER THREE

Diseases of the Drugs in Type 2 Diabetes

How are you doing? We've gotten through all the "diseases of the drugs" of hypertension and dyslipidemia. Now we're rounding the corner into type 2 diabetes.

Maybe let's both get a mug of herbal tea. Fabulous idea, my dear Reader!

There! That's better, huh? Let's dive in…

The Drugs That Can Cause Type 2 Diabetes—Your Potential Past

Since you've been reading this book like a novel, if you've been medicated for high blood pressure or cholesterol issues, you may now suspect that your recently diagnosed diabetes has something to do with your past prescriptions. You're probably right!

Blood pressure-lowering medications from several classes can *cause* type 2 diabetes. **Loop diuretics, thiazide diuretics** and **beta blockers** are all implicated—and so is **clonidine**. Clonidine is used more in children with ADD/ADHD than in adults with high blood pressure these days. Crazily enough, the seven-year-old kid with ADD gets the same dose as the fifty-seven-year-old adult with hypertension.

Lipid-lowering medication also pushes folks into type 2 diabetes. The **statins** have become rather infamous for this, ever since the class action suit against the manufacturer of Lipitor (the branded version of **atorvastatin**). **Niacin** can also cause type 2 diabetes when dosed at pharmacological levels. This typically happens when treating cholesterol problems "naturally."

(Did you get your answer? Are you one of the way-too-many people with medication-induced diabetes? I'll still ask that you make lifestyle changes in the flip side of this book—if you want "medical miracles," that is!)

Remember in the chapter on hypertension how I mentioned that medications used to affect the heart positively usually do something negative to the lungs, and vice versa? The **beta agonists**, short-acting and long-acting, that are used for allergies, asthma, exercise-induced bronchospasms, emphysema, chronic bronchitis, and often short-term for respiratory infections, can cause blood glucose to be so high as to warrant more medication. Asthmatics, know that **theophylline** and **epinephrine** can raise blood sugar levels as well.

Lithium and **"mood stabilizers"**—these are actually anti-psychotics and anti-epileptic medications being used to stabilize mood in depression to avoid the high potential of the antidepressant causing bipolar 2 disorder—can cause type 2 diabetes. (Please check **Appendix C, Table 1** for the list. "Mood stabilizers" are being used for all kinds of things they've not gotten approval for. These will be covered at length in a future book. You might very well be taking one of these agents under the guise of something altogether different.)

Hormones, steroids, and fluoroquinolone antibiotics (ciprofloxacin, levofloxacin, moxifloxacin) can all cause hyperglycemia. (Note: The fluoroquinolones can also cause hypoglycemia—*low* blood glucose!)

Medications for **depression or anxiety**, sometimes used for smoking cessation and/or sleep, can cause fluctuations in blood glucose, landing patients in the diabetic range. (Again, please check Appendix C, Table 1 for the complete list. This is another group of medications frequently prescribed for off-label use.)

Here's a twist: **Monoclonal antibodies** ("MABs"/biologics) being used for auto-immune conditions (mostly), including cancer, can cause type 1 diabetes **and** type 2 diabetes. Type 1 diabetes is an autoimmune form of diabetes.

*Wait. The "MABs" are used to treat autoimmune conditions, right? Yet they can **cause** more autoimmunity?*

Yes, they can. It's a complex topic, but once one autoimmune condition has taken place, the patient is at a much higher risk for additional autoimmune conditions to develop. The "MABs" manufacturers explain this by saying their agents merely uncover latent (hidden) issues. What patients are saying is that they didn't have type 1 diabetes—or tuberculosis or cancer or JC virus or systemic lupus erythematosus, etc.—until they got put on a biologic for something else.

The **retinoids** that people use for acne and wrinkles can cause type 2 diabetes.

Anti-retrovirals in the protease inhibitor family, used to treat HIV/AIDS, can also cause type 2 diabetes. As a matter of fact, patients who have HIV often die now of cardiovascular disease in the form of high blood pressure, dyslipidemia, and type 2 diabetes rather than AIDS!

The Secondary Diagnoses That Taking Drugs To Manage Type 2 Diabetes Can Cause—Your Potential Present/Future

There are *nine* (9) categories of drugs used to treat type 2 diabetes. This is a lifestyle-driven disease, having less to do with your genes and far more to do with how you learned to prepare and eat food from your family of origin or from those who chose to raise you.

We discussed this earlier, but it bears repeating. We have control over somewhere between 70 percent (what I was taught in school, twenty-plus years ago) and 92 percent (what I learned mere weeks ago) of how our genes express themselves. That means our genes are "locked" at only 8 to

30 percent! Our genes determine how tall we can grow, but not that we'll absolutely grow that tall. Genes decide what color our eyes and hair will be naturally. Genes determine our birth gender.

Our genes have a suggested destination for us, but for the most part, *we* get to determine our paths in life. Much of our chosen path is determined by how we choose to feed ourselves!

Our choices include more than the food and drink we consume. I'm talking about the rest of our consumerism habits as well: the music we listen to, the books and magazines we read, the movies we watch, and the friends we choose. All these factors definitely influence how our genes express themselves.

When we're old enough to spend time with other families, we start to compare and contrast the friends' families with our own. That's when we start making bigger decisions on our own, too, like habits of hygiene, clothing, and whether we take lunch to school or eat the cafeteria food.

I am assuming (*Oh, boy!*) that, because you are reading this book, your basic needs are being met. You have a safe living space that provides shelter and protection and you have "food security"—sufficient funds to buy food. Not everyone has these basics. You, my friend, are privileged to grow beyond the constraints of your upbringing. You have the *freedom to choose* how you will live. We are presented with choices at every turn.

If you didn't know that high blood pressure was a consequence of life choices, now you do.

If you didn't know that cholesterol abnormalities were a lifestyle issue, now you do.

If you didn't know that type 2 diabetes was an expression of your genes *because of your personal choices,* now you do!

"Knowing is half the battle!" — G.I. Joe

Every one of these "problems" is there, I believe, to teach you something valuable about what poet Mary Oliver called "your one, wild and precious life." The lesson is that you are in charge of *you*. No one else has that power unless you turn it over to another, abdicating your own volition.

You are ever so much more than the sum of your parts! There will literally never be another you on this planet. Please, take excellent care of *you*—as if you were your oldest, best, most constant friend, who speaks to you in the kindest way possible that will still get your attention. That's what your physical body is to your soul/spirit.

I've mentioned earlier that medical management does not stop the progression of disease. I've also mentioned that the manufacturers of anti-diabetic medications, anti-hypertensive medications, and anti-cholesterol medications *all* state that their drugs should be used *in conjunction with diet/ lifestyle changes.*

The **sulfonylureas, alpha-glucosidase inhibitors, meglitinides** (aka "glinides"), and **dipeptidyl peptase-4 (DPP-4) inhibitors** are indicated for use only in adults with type 2 diabetes. Same with the **thiazolidinediones**, both of which have been removed from other world markets for causing congestive heart failure and associated deaths. Rosiglitazone has been pulled from the UK, India, New Zealand and South America; pioglitazone has been prohibited in France and Germany. Yet both these drugs remain available in the US market.

One **biguanide**, metformin hydrochloride, is indicated for use in adults and pediatric patients ten years of age and older with type 2 diabetes mellitus.

Did you catch that? Ten years of age and older. Diabetes used to be the "affluent older white man's disease"—because the guy who'd successfully climbed the corporate ladder had the luxury of what money could buy, namely sweets, alcohol, cigars, and red meat. But now we're medicating our children for this absolutely preventable and reversible disease.

As newer drugs for diabetes have entered the marketplace, additional indications have been granted them besides improving glycemic control in adults and children. **The glucagon-like peptide receptor-1 (GLP1) agonists** showcase these additional uses, along with the progression of disease despite medical management. Watch closely.

Exenatide, lixisenatide, and dulaglutide hold indications for use only in type 2 diabetes. The cousins liraglutide, semaglutide and tirzepatide have indications for use in type 2 diabetes *and* obesity. Same drug, same dose, same manufacturer; different warnings and precautions. More on that theme in the next few pages.

Dulaglutide also gets the added indication for reducing the risk of major adverse cardiovascular events (cardiovascular death, non-fatal myocardial infarction, or non-fatal stroke) in adults with type 2 diabetes mellitus who have established cardiovascular disease or multiple cardiovascular risk factors.

Semaglutide has the additional indications to reduce the risk of major adverse cardiovascular events and to reduce the risk of sustained eGFR decline, end-stage kidney disease, and cardiovascular death in adults with type 2 diabetes mellitus and chronic kidney disease.

Kidney disease. That's a complication or continuation of type 2 diabetes, right? Yes. So are the major cardiovascular events. The disease process continues to progress despite medication.

So, even at this point, changes for health could stop all this sequelae of the original diagnosis? You got it, my dear Reader!

The **sodium-glucose co-transporter type-2 (SGLT-2) inhibitors** use very similar language, but through the lens of end-stage kidney disease.

Reading this now through the lens of diabetes progression... This is just so sad! It may become outrageously unacceptable in your mind before long.

So far, we've looked at eight categories of drugs to try, alter, and combine prior to adding insulin injections. After insulin is implemented, there's the **amylin analog** pramlintide. This is an add-on to a type-1 or type-2 diabetic's insulin when blood sugar remains uncontrolled.

Nine categories of drugs, plus insulin injections. For type 2 diabetes.

That's rather absurd! I know, right?

And because these agents don't change the disease process—only changes to diet and exercise and sleep and thoughts and emotions and beliefs (i.e., *lifestyle*) can change **lifestyle-driven diseases**—the newer agents on the market are combinations of metformin + glipizide, rosiglitazone + glimepiride, pioglitazone + metformin, empagliflozin + linagliptin + metformin.

Three different agents? Yes, my dear Reader, three different agents. Because if a little worked a bit, a lot must work much better. Only it doesn't. The disease continues to progress.

Your hemoglobin A1c reading measures your average blood sugar levels over a three-month period, so it's useful as a measure of diabetic disease and how effective treatment might be. A healthy number is less than 5.7 percent. Anything over 6 is considered diabetic.

Individually, drugs to treat diabetes only lower the number by ½ to 2 points. That's fine if your number is 7.9 and you can get it down to 5.9. But what if your number is 17.9? That's why doctors sometimes prescribe triple-combination drugs; still, those can only go so far.

Here's the kicker, taken from the glyburide monograph, but added to every anti-diabetic category but one:

> "Macrovascular Outcomes: There have been no clinical studies establishing conclusive evidence of macrovascular risk reduction with glyburide tablets or any other anti-diabetic drug."

Macrovascular means *big vessels*. The statement above is saying that, despite taking this drug to lower your blood sugar numbers, there's no evidence that you'll be spared a heart attack or stroke. In fact, your risk of an adverse macrovascular event may be higher while on a sulfonylurea. That's the *Special Warning* on the class of sulfonylureas.

The medications are given to, hopefully, provide *microvascular* risk reduction. Microvascular means *little vessels*: the blood vessels in your retina, kidneys, genitalia, fingers and toes. The SGLT-2 inhibitors showed a wee bit of *macrovascular* protection (although it's not clinically significant), so they got the green light to go to market. However, the *microvascular* risk reduction is gone. Patients taking canagliflozin have an *increased risk of lower limb amputation!* This was a *Boxed Warning* until 2020 when it was downgraded to a mere "warning."

Yikes!

But I've jumped ahead of myself. Let's start at the chronological beginning and work our way into present-day medical management for type 2 diabetes.

If one of the **sulfonylureas** is your current anti-diabetes medication, the most problematic concern is the special warning of increased risk in adverse macrovascular events (heart attack, stroke). It's harder to drop excess weight while on a sulfonylurea. Hypoglycemia (low blood sugar) can be a risk on sulfonylureas, so get in the habit of checking your blood glucose routinely. Average drop in HbA1c with sulfonylureas is 1 to 2 percent.

If you're taking **metformin**—which catapulted into popularity on the heels of the research that shed the "special warning" light on the sulfonylureas—you probably won't be surprised about the very common adverse effect of diarrhea. In fact, you've probably experienced the metformin-induced loose bowel syndrome. Many doctors will raise the dose of metformin until it causes the uncomfortable, unpredictable, and unappealing diarrhea. Metformin also carries the *Boxed Warning* of potentially deadly lactic acidosis. Because of its subtle onset and nonspecific set of symptoms—a generalized sensation of feeling "unwell," muscle pains, abdominal pain, and sleepiness—this condition can progress without medical follow-up until it becomes critical. The potential for dangerously low blood glucose levels is compounded if metformin is used along with a sulfonylurea. The average drop in HbA1c with metformin is 1 to 2 percent.

The **alpha-glucosidase inhibitors** never gained traction in the marketplace, probably because they caused a reduction in HbA1c of a mere half percentage point. The side effects include abdominal pain, diarrhea, and flatulence. Post-marketing, there have been accounts of rare fulminant hepatitis (fatal), and pneumatosis cystoides intestinalis, a condition of severe and life-threatening intestinal torsion. (*That's a tongue-twister!* It's literally an intestinal twister, Reader.)

Thiazolidinediones come with the *Boxed Warning* of causing or worsening congestive heart failure, and each has been banned in other world markets. They can also cause bladder cancer, liver failure, bone fractures, macular edema, and lower limb swelling. Average drop in HbA1c with thiazolidinediones is 1 to 1.5 percent.

The **meglitinides** are not to be paired with NPH insulin. They have no *Boxed Warning* but can cause hypoglycemia. (Yes, a drop in blood glucose is exactly what's wanted, but too much of a good thing can often yield bad outcomes. Monitor your blood sugar routinely!) Average drop in HbA1c with meglitinides is 1 to 1.5 percent.

The class that's overtaking the marketplace these days, for weight loss and type 2 diabetes, is the **glucagon-like peptide receptor-1 (GLP-1) agonists**. Who *hasn't* heard of Ozempic? Sheesh! These do have a *Boxed Warning* for causing thyroid C-cell tumors and medullary thyroid cancer. The regular warnings and precautions vary only slightly between the agents. All of them warn of acute pancreatitis, acute kidney injury, severe GI disease (a class action suit is underway), immunogenicity, gallbladder disease, diabetic retinopathy, hypoglycemia, and pulmonary aspiration during deep sedation or anesthesia. I suspect "Ozempic face/butt" will soon be added to the list, only in medicalized language. The GLP-1 agonists lower A1c by an average of only 1 percent.

When these agents are used for weight loss, they get a couple of other warnings: heart rate increase and suicidal behavior and ideation. Same drug, same dose, same manufacturer; different set of warnings. Curious, don't you think? As a side note, any deviation in healthy blood glucose—too high or too low—can push a person into depression and/or anxiety.

The **amylin analog** pramlintide has a *Boxed Warning* for severe hypoglycemia. This medication is prescribed for certain patients meeting exacting criteria and already using insulin, yet it only yields a 0.4 to 0.6 percent drop in HbA1c.

Scoring only slightly higher with a HbA1c drop of 0.8 percent are the **dipeptidyl peptase-4 (DPP-4) inhibitors**. They should not be used in tandem with either insulin or a sulfonylurea due to subsequent risk of hypoglycemia. No *Boxed Warning* yet, but DPP-4 inhibitors increase the risk of pancreatitis, heart failure, acute kidney failure, severe arthralgias, and a serious skin condition called bullous pemphigoid.

Last, but not least are the **sodium-glucose co-transporter type-2 (SGLT-2) inhibitors**. These are the agents that supposedly offer a smidgeon of *macrovascular* risk reduction. Canagliflozin (one agent in this class) had a *Boxed Warning* for increased risk of limb amputations! That got reduced to a "regular" warning in 2020—many bizarre occurrences transpired in medicine that year—along with a warning of volume depletion with severe drops in blood pressure, ketoacidosis, bone fractures, increased LDL cholesterol, urosepsis (significant infection starting in the urinary tract and spreading elsewhere), pyelonephritis (inflammatory infection inside the kidney—typically starting from the bladder), kidney injury (one can see the progression), and genital fungal infections to the point of "necrotizing fasciitis"—a flesh-eating infection of the "private parts."

Y'all, I can't make this stuff up! These agents should not be paired with insulin or sulfonylureas due to the risk of hypoglycemia. On their own, they decrease HbA1c 0.6 to 1.2 percent.

Nutritional Deficiencies Commonly Seen In Patients With Type 2 Diabetes—Your Potential Future

This section is shorter than the rest found in this book, as many of these classes are not yet known to cause nutritional deficiencies.

The sulfonylureas waste coenzyme Q-10 and magnesium. CoQ-10 is a necessary cofactor in the mitochondria of cells to turn ADP into ATP. Without it, expect physical and mental fatigue with poor concentration, memory lapses, and "negative" mood changes.

Magnesium in the body is distributed approximately distributed 60 percent in bone, 25 percent in muscles, with the rest in soft tissues and fluids (gastric). Insufficient magnesium can cause fatigue, irritability, weakness, muscle tightness/spasms, dysmenorrhea, hypertension, cardiomyopathy, nerve conduction problems, anorexia, insomnia, sugar cravings, poor nail growth, and anxiety.

Metformin wastes folate and vitamin B12. A folate deficiency can show up as poor growth, megaloblastic anemia, glossitis, or GI tract disturbances.

A vitamin B12 deficiency is a different kind of anemia: pernicious anemia and accompanying progressive peripheral neuropathy with pronounced anemia. There's also fatigue, depression, confusion, memory loss, psychosis, glossitis, achlorhydria (insufficient gastric acid), impaired lymphocyte response (decreased immune system response), decreased phagocyte and PMN response (deeper, more decreased immune system response), spinal degeneration, and macrocytic cells (really large cells—part of the "look" of pernicious anemia).

Diabetics as a class of patients tend to be low in magnesium, chromium, and zinc; possibly also biotin, potassium, and copper. The full list, along with best food options from which to obtain these vitally important nutrients, is in Appendix C, Table 3.

The Other Ingredients Found In Anti-Diabetic Drugs

Every drug has fillers or excipients in it. Supplements are often just as loaded as the pharmaceuticals. Granted, not every filler is inherently evil; but if I'm going to ask my patients/clients to take a product every day, maybe several times a day, over a prolonged period of time, I really want every ingredient to count toward health, not disease. I ask that you continue to read along with me and draw your own conclusions about these ingredients commonly found in anti-diabetic drugs:

Carboxymethylcellulose calcium: Calcium salt of carboxymethylcellulose, commercially made from wood, chemically modified.

Polyethylene glycol, polyvinyl alcohol, polyvinylpyrrolidone, propylene glycol, polysorbate 80.... If I need to consult a chemist to know what an ingredient actually is, I get suspicious. Why are these necessary? I teach my patients/clients to put back on the shelf products with ingredients they cannot pronounce and choose something "real" instead.

Polysorbate 80: Contamination concerns: ethylene dioxide, a known human carcinogen, unsafe for use in cosmetics, known respiratory toxicant, limited evidence of kidney toxicity, eye/lung/skin irritant, strong evidence of human immune toxicant; *Unacceptable* per EWG.

1,4-dioxane: a synthetic industrial material, completely miscible in water, unstable at higher temperatures/pressure, explosive with prolonged exposure to light/air, resistant to biodegradation, likely to be carcinogenic, upper respiratory, kidney and liver damage.) https://www.epa.gov/sites/default/files/2014-03/documents/ffrro_factsheet_contaminant_14-dioxane_january2014_final.pdf

Triacetin, titanium dioxide, ammonium hydroxide, and sodium hydroxide—also commonly found in anti-diabetic medications—are all "expected to be harmful or toxic."

Things I'd expect, like corn starch and sugar, also are in pills for diabetics. I wonder if they're genetically modified. Most of the corn grown in the US is GMO (94 percent), as is sugar (95 percent). Personally, I'm cutting back on my GMO intake because glyphosate (brand name "RoundUp") poisoning is all too common in humans.

Other sweeteners—like glycerin, mannitol, and meglumine—are in many anti-diabetic prescription pills. The last two are sugar alcohols, so they're non-caloric, but I am a recovering sugar addict! *Why* are sweeteners used in pills? Metformin has artificial blackberry flavoring added to the pill. Who is sucking the coating off these pills? That's a great lure for a small child, but for adults? And the sweeteners in medication lead to more accidental ingestion by children. Iron poisoning happens frequently with children who associate their brightly colored and good-tasting chewable multivitamin with candy; if left to their own unattended devices, kids will eat the entire content of that multivitamin container.

FD&C colors, with and without the "lake" in the name, often carry the danger of adherence to heavy metals, typically aluminum. These contaminants can cause concerns over cancer and neurotoxicity. *I'm concerned!*

I get it. But the medications contain only a tiny amount of these potentially problematic ingredients. What's the big deal?

How do deep canyons happen? They can be formed by shifts in the earth's crust, essentially pulling land masses apart. They can be formed by a massive amount of water (like a global flood over a few months), the force of which breaks open the earth. They can also be formed by the constant wearing down of rock over time by water and wind (like a river twisting through rock over thousands of years).

The big deal is that sick people being given medications laced with ingredients that can make people sick seems a dreadful idea to me—especially when these ingredients become a daily assault to the exquisite design of the human being in the name of "better health."

You've read the risks. You've started, at least, to count the costs that aren't strictly financial. *You are the Big Deal, Reader!* I, for one, want better for you.

When I point out problems that I see in the world around me, I typically offer potential solutions. Disease is plucking my nerves, Readers. I'm sick of watching beautiful, brilliant, creative humans suffer needlessly and die before fulfilling their purposes on this planet. It's one thing to be ignorant—unaware and uninformed, but it's another to be informed and willfully irresponsible. The real kicker is, we get *to choose.*

Are you, like me, sick and tired of being sick and tired? If you believe that knowledge is power once put into personal, practical application—and if you are ready to live in the fullness of life that is available to us all—flip this book over now.

Let's walk through the processes of **reversing** these lifestyle-driven diseases called hypertension, dyslipidemia and type 2 diabetes.

How fun! I haven't had a flip-book since I was a kid! ☺

APPENDIX A

Hypertension

Table 1: Drugs that can cause hypertension

Table 2: Drugs used to manage hypertension, warnings/precautions, efficacy, nutrients wasted

Table 3: Nutrient deficiencies caused by the drugs used to manage hypertension, food sources

Table 4: Other ingredients in drugs used to manage hypertension

Blood Pressure Log

TABLE 1: Drugs that can raise blood pressure, risking the diagnosis of hypertension.

Drug name, generic	Drug name, brand	Drug class	Indications for use
Albuterol Levalbuterol	Ventolin, Proventil, ProAir Xopenex	Short acting beta-2 agonists; bronchodilators	Bronchospasm; albuterol also is indicated for use in exercise-induced bronchospasm
Formoterol (+budesonide) Salmeterol (+fluticasone)	Forodil, Perforomist (Symbicort) Serevent (Advair, AirDuo)	Long acting beta-2 agonists; bronchodilators	Asthma, COPD (chronic obstructive pulmonary disease, such as emphysema and chronic bronchitis), exercise-induced bronchospasm
Theophylline	TheoDur, Theocron, Theo-24, Elixophyllin	Methylxanthine; bronchodilator	Asthma, COPD
Lithium	Eskalith, Lithobid	Anti-mania	Bipolar disorder (age seven years and older)
Aripiprazole Risperidone Olanzapine Ziprasidone Quetiapine Lurasidone Clozapine	Abilify Risperdal, Perseris Zyprexa Geodon Seroquel Latuda Clozaril, FasaClo, Versacloz	Anti-psychotics, often called "mood stabilizers"	Schizophrenia; some also have approval for use in major depressive disorder, bipolar disorder, suicidal behavior in schizophrenia or schizoaffective disorder, irritability in autism, bipolar mania, Tourette's disorder
Gabapentin Phenytoin Lamotrigine Divalproex	Neurontin, Gralise Dilantin Lamictal Depakote	Anticonvulsants or anti-epileptics, often called "mood stabilizers"	Partial (focal) seizures; others are indicated for use in nerve pain after shingles, generalized seizures, status epilepticus, bipolar disorder, mania, migraines

APPENDIX A: Hypertension

Drug name, generic	Drug name, brand	Drug class	Indications for use
Prednisone	Deltasone	Corticosteroids	Anti-inflammatory or immune suppressant agents across most body systems and conditions: allergic, neoplastic, skin, blood, gut, eyes, joints, skin, immune, nervous, endocrine, respiratory, kidney; solid organ rejection. Used by mouth, applied to the skin, inhaled into the nose or mouth, or injected.
Beclomethasone	Qvar		
Hydrocortisone	Cortef, Solu-Cortef		
Dexamethasone	Decadron		
Methylprednisolone	Medrol		
Prednisolone	Oropred, Millipred		
Triamcinolone	Kenalog		
Budesonide	Pulmocort		
Medroxyprogesterone	Provera, Depo-Provera	Progestins	Contraception and heavy menstrual bleeding; medroxyprogesterone is also indicated for use in lack of menstrual bleeding, endometriosis, endometrial overgrowth and cancer.
Levonorgestrel (found in mini-pills, combo contraceptives, IUDs, "day after" pills)	Mirena, Lyletta, Skyla, Kyleena; Plan B, Next Choice, My Way, React, Option 2, Aftera		

Diseases of the Drugs

Drug name, generic	Drug name, brand	Drug class	Indications for use
Estrone	Kestrone-5, Estragyn/LA 5, EstroneAQ, Aquest	Estrogens	Peri/post-menopausal symptoms, various cancers, bHRT, atrophic urethritis and vaginitis, dyspareunia, primary ovarian failure, HRT, contraception, abnormal uterine bleeding, gender dysphoria
Estradiol	Estrace, Estradiol Patch, Climara, Vagifem, Estring, Imvexxy		
Estriol	Ovestin, Evelon, Femastin, Gynest		
Ethinyl estradiol			
Conjugated estrogens	Premarin, Cenestin, Enjuvia		
Estropipate	Ogen, Ortho-Est		
Diethylstilbestrol	Stilphostrol		
Testosterone	Androderm, AndroGel, Fortesta, Testim, Depo-Testosterone, Testopel, Aveed, Natesto, Vogelxo, Xyosted, Jatenzo, Tlando, Kyzatrex	Androgens, anabolic steroids	Primary hypogonadism, hypogonadotropic hypogonadism; certain cancers
Methyltestosterone	Methitest, Testred		
Modafinil	Provigil	Central nervous system stimulants (unknown class)	Narcolepsy, obstructive sleep apnea, shift work sleep disorder.
Armodafinil	Nuvigil		

APPENDIX A: Hypertension

Drug name, generic	Drug name, brand	Drug class	Indications for use
Amitriptyline (hyper/hypotension)	Elavil	Anti-depressants, tricyclics	Major depressive disorder; some have indications for use in bipolar disorder, sleep issues, anxiety, bed-wetting
Desipramine	Norpramin		
Doxepin	Sinequan, Silenor		
Notriptyline	Pamelor		
Venlafaxine	Effexor	Anti-depressants, serotonin and norepinephrine reuptake inhibitors (SNRI)	Major depressive disorder; some agents have indications for use in generalized anxiety disorder, panic disorder, social anxiety disorder, fibromyalgia, chronic pain, nerve pain associated with diabetes
Desvenlafaxine	Pristiq, Khedezla		
Duloxetine	Cymbalta, Drizalma		
Milnacipran	Savella		
Levomilnacipran	Fetzima		
Fluoxetine	Prozac, Serafem	Anti-depressants, selective serotonin reuptake inhibitors (SSRI)	Major depressive disorder (excluding Serafem which is approved for pre-menstrual dysphoric disorder only); many are indicated for use in bipolar major depression, bulimia nervosa, obsessive compulsive disorder, panic disorder, treatment resistant depression, social anxiety disorder, pre-menstrual dysphoric disorder, post-traumatic stress disorder
Paroxetine	Paxil, Pexeva, Brisdelle		
Citalopram	Celexa		
Fluvoxamine	Luvox (approved only for obsessive compulsive disorder)		
Trazodone	Desyrel	Anti-depressant, serotonin antagonist and reuptake inhibitor (SARI)	Major depressive disorder
Bupropion/XL	Wellbutrin/XL, Zyban, Aplenzin, Forfivo	Anti-depressant, norepinephrine and dopamine reuptake inhibitor (NDRI)	Major depressive disorder (all brands but Zyban which is indicated for smoking cessation), seasonal affective disorder (Aplenzin and Wellbutrin XL)

Diseases of the Drugs

Drug name, generic	Drug name, brand	Drug class	Indications for use
Tranylcypromine	**Parnate--Boxed Warning: hypertensive crisis**	Anti-depressants, monoamine oxidase inhibitor (MAOI)	Major depressive disorder
Ibuprofen	Advil, Motrin	Non-steroidal anti-inflammatory drugs (NSAIDs)	Inflammatory diseases and disorders, pain (some indicated for acute, some indicated for chronic, some indicated for auto-immune), fever reduction
Naproxen	Naprosyn, Alleve, Anaprox		
Indomethacin	Indocin, Tyvorbex		
Piroxicam	Feldene		
Meloxicam	Mobic		
Oxaprozin	DayPro		
Nabumetone	Relafen		
Ketorolac	Toradol		
Ketoprofen	Orudis, Oruvail		
Etodolac	Lodine		
Diflunisal	Dolobid		
Celecoxib	Celebrex		
Selegiline	Eldepryl, Emsam, Zelapar	Anti-Parkinson's agents, MAOIs	Parkinson's disease (PD) (Selegiline: PD & Major Depressive Disorder)
Rasagiline	Azilect		

APPENDIX A: Hypertension

Drug name, generic	Drug name, brand	Drug class	Indications for use
Amphetamine	Adzenys, Dynavel, Evekeo	Central nervous system stimulants	Attention deficit/hyperactivity disorder; some have indications for use in weight loss, narcolepsy, binge-eating disorder
Dextroamphetamine	Dexedrine, ProCentra, Zenzedi		
Lysdexamfetamine	Vyvanse		
Methylphenidate	Concerta, Quillivant, Ritalin, Daytrana, Aptensio, Methylin		
Dexmethylphenidate	Focalin		
Atomoxetine	Strattera	Selective nor-epinephrine reuptake inhibitor (the other SNRI)	Attention deficit/hyperactivity disorder
Caffeine	In coffee, tea (black, green, oolong, pu'erh), pills (Even the decaf versions contain caffeine!)	Legal, widely available central nervous system stimulant	
Methamphetamine Cocaine PCP MDMA/ecstasy/molly		Illegal street drugs ("uppers")	
Pseudoephedrine	Sudafed, Contact Cold (many)	Alpha/beta receptor agonist; Non-selective alpha receptor agonist	Over-the-counter decongestants (pills and eye/nasal sprays)
Phenylephrine	Sudafed-PE, Neo-Synephrine (many)		

Diseases of the Drugs

Drug name, generic	Drug name, brand	Drug class	Indications for use
Sumatriptan	Imitrex	Serotonin 5-HT1 receptor agonists, "triptans"	Anti-migraine medication (pills, nasal sprays)
Eletriptan	Relpax		
Naratriptan	Amerge		
Almotriptan	Axert		
Frovatriptan	Frova		
Rizatriptan	Maxalt		
Zolmitriptan	Zomig		
Acetaminophen (paracetamol)	Tylenol (many)	Over-the-counter pain reliever	Mild to moderate pain, fever reduction
Mycophenolate mofetil	Cellcept	Various kinds of immune suppressants	Kidney, heart, liver transplants; autoimmune conditions, including certain cancers
Cyclosporine	Sandimmune		
Adalimumab	Humira		*can cause hypotension OR hypertension (cardiac collapse, myocardial infarction, etc)
Bevacizumab	Avastin		
Cetuximab	Erbitux		
Ipilimumab*	Yervoy		
Ramucirumab	Cyramza		
Rituximab*	Rituxan		
Trastuzumab*	Herceptin		
Certolizumab	Cimzia		
Golimumab	Simponi		
Tocilizumab	Actemra		
Basiliximab	Simulect		

APPENDIX A: Hypertension

Drug name, generic	Drug name, brand	Drug class	Indications for use
Tretinoin (hypo/hypertension)	Vesanoid, Retin-A, Altreno, Stieva-A	Retinoids	Acne, acute promyelocytic leukemia, necrobiosis lipoidica diabeticorum, photoaging of skin, and lichen sclerosis; skin lesions caused by cutaneous T-cell lymphoma+
Bexarotene+	Targretin		
Tipranavir	Aptivus	Anti-retrovirals, protease inhibitors	Used in the treatment of HIV and AIDS
Atazanavir	Reyataz		
Atazanavir/cobicistat	Evotaz		
Lopinavir/ritonavir	Kaletra		
Fosamprenavir	Lexiva		
Ritonavir	Norvir		
Darunavir	Prezista		
Darunavir/cobicistat	Prezcobix		

https://www.cancer.gov/about-cancer/treatment/types/immunotherapy/monoclonal-antibodies#what-are-the-side-effects-of-monoclonal-antibodies AND https://www.singlecare.com/drug-classes/monoclonal-antibodies

Table 2: Below are the drugs currently used to *treat/manage* hypertension. The average drop in blood pressure is also listed where found. ("Normal" = 120/80 or lower; 130+ systolic or 80+ diastolic on more than one occasion, in office, is considered high blood pressure.)

DRUG CLASS: Thiazide diuretics

DRUG NAMES, Generic	DRUG NAMES, Brand	NUTRIENTS DEPLETED	BW; Precautions; Populations
Hydrochlorothiazide	Microzide, HydroDiuril, Esidrix	*CoQ-10* *Magnesium* *Potassium* *Calcium* *Sodium* *Zinc* *Vitamin D* (BP reduction not listed)	Loss of sodium and potassium; "latent diabetes may become manifest;" glaucoma, myopia, choroidal effusion. Activation/exacerbation of SLE. Caution in patients with renal/liver disease, allergy, asthma. Avoid with lithium. Do not interchange Mykrox/Zaroxolyn!
Chlorothiazide	Diuril		
Indapamide	Lozol		
Metolazone	Mykrox, Zaroxolyn		
Chlorthalidone	Thalitone		

DRUG CLASS: Loop Diuretics

DRUG NAMES, Generic	DRUG NAMES, Brand	NUTRIENTS DEPLETED	BW; Precautions; Populations
Furosemide	Lasix	*CoQ10* *Magnesium* *Potassium* *Calcium* *Sodium* *Zinc* *Vitamins B (1,6,12)* *Vitamin C* *Folic Acid (folate)* *Mixed tocopherols (vitamin E)* *Phosphorus* BP reduction not listed	Titrate to patient; monitor; ototoxicity. Hypokalemia, ototoxicity. **Bumetanide can cause profound diuresis.** Hypotension, worsening renal function, electrolyte imbalances, ototoxicity.
Bumetanide	Bumex		
Torsemide	Demadex, Soaanz		

APPENDIX A: Hypertension

DRUG CLASS: Potassium-sparing diuretics

DRUG NAMES, Generic	DRUG NAMES, Brand	NUTRIENTS DEPLETED	BW; Precautions; Populations
Spironolactone	Aldactone		Avoid in Addison's.
Eplerenone*	Inspra	*6-13/3-7	*Avoid in diabetics, patients with severe kidney disease.
Triamterene^	Dyrenium	Folate, calcium, zinc (triamterene)	^Avoid in severe kidney/liver diseae, urination problems. **Triamterene can cause dangerously high potassium.**
Amiloride+	Midamor		+Avoid in patients with acidosis or urination problems.

DRUG CLASS: Alpha-2 agonists

DRUG NAMES, Generic	DRUG NAMES, Brand	NUTRIENTS DEPLETED	BW; Precautions; Populations
Clonidine	Catapres (Kapvay)	16/12	(First two listed are also used in kids with ADD/ADHD)
Guanfacine	Tenex (Intuniv)		
Methyldopa*	Aldomet	13/8.4 No known nutrient depletions	**Do NOT abruptly discontinue!**

DRUG CLASS: Alpha-1 antagonists

DRUG NAMES, Generic	DRUG NAMES, Brand	NUTRIENTS DEPLETED	BW; Precautions; Populations
Doxazosin	Cardura/XL, Cascor	9-10/5-8 No known nutrient depletions	Cardura XL for BPH **Do NOT abruptly discontinue!**
Prazosin	Doxadura, Carduran, Minipress		
Terazosin	Hytrin		

DRUG CLASS: Beta-blockers

DRUG NAMES, Generic	DRUG NAMES, Brand	NUTRIENTS DEPLETED	BW; Precautions; Populations
Atenolol	Tenormin	11/12	First generation: non-selective, affecting heart, kidneys, lungs, GI tract, liver, uterus, vascular smooth muscle, skeletal muscle
Propranolol+	Inderal, InnoPran	*CoQ-10*	
Nadolol	Corgard	*Melatonin*	
Timolol maleate	Blocadren	*Chromium*	
Penbutolol sulfate*	Levatol		
Sotalol HCl@	Betapace	AFIB/AFL	**@VT/AFIB/AFL**
Pindolol*	Visken	Glaucoma	*Intrinsic Sympathomimetic Activity
Labetalol HCl^	Trandate, Normodyne	7.5-9/3.5-5.5	Second generation: B2 specific, affecting mostly the heart
Metoprolol	Lopressor, Toprol XL		+Quinidine-like (anesthetic-like) action
Acebutolol HCl*+	Sectral		
Bisoprolol fumarate	Zebeta		^Block B and A1-receptors, increasing peripheral vasodilation
Esmolol HCl	Brevibloc		**Abrupt discontinuation may cause exacerbation of angina and/or MI!**
Betaxolol HCl+	Kerlone		Ramp up, taper down dose.
Carvedilol^	Coreg		*Greater clearance in Black patients; likely less effective.*

APPENDIX A: Hypertension

DRUG CLASS: Calcium-channel blockers

DRUG NAMES, Generic	DRUG NAMES, Brand	NUTRIENTS DEPLETED	BW; Precautions; Populations
Amlodipine	Norvasc, Norliqva, Katerzia	12/6	Angina, MI, edema. *Better option (monotherapy) for Black patients; risk of gingival hyperplasia** **Procardia capsules should not be used for the acute reduction of blood pressure, nor for the control of essential hypertension, nor within the first week or two after myocardial infarction, and they should also be avoided in the setting of acute coronary syndrome (when infarction may be imminent).** NOTE: Many of these products contain PEG (+parabens, colorants, corn, pork, talc, magnesium stearate, et.al.) *Monitor Potassium in all!*
Felodipine*	Plendil	12-19/6-8	
Nisoldipine	Sular	12-13/6-7 *Amlodipine: Potassium Vitamin D Diltiazem, Nifedipine, Verapamil.*	
Isradipine	Dynacirc/CR		
Levamlodipine	Conjupri		
Nicardipine	Cardene/SR, Nifediac CC		
Nifedipine	Afeditab/CR, Adalat/CC, Procardia/XL, Nifedical XL	2.6-10.6/5.1-10.6	
Diltiazem	Cardizem/CD/LA Cartia XT, Tiazac, Dilt-XR, Taztia XT, Dilacor XR, Tiadylt ER, Matzim LA, Diltzac, Diltia XT		
Verapamil	Calan/SR, Covera HS, Verelan/PM		

DRUG CLASS: Angiotensin Converting Enzyme (ACE) inhibitors

DRUG NAMES, Generic	DRUG NAMES, Brand	NUTRIENTS DEPLETED	BW; Precautions; Populations
Lisinopril	Zestril, Prinivil, Qbrelis	*Sodium* *Zinc*	**Fetal and neonatal morbidity and mortality.**
Enalapril	Vasotec, Epened	6/4	
Ramipril	Altace	6-12/4-7	Malignancies, Renal Failure, Hyperkalemia, Angioedema, Neutropenia, Hepatic Failure. Less benefit in Black patients, greater risk of angioedema; cough that may affect performers, speakers
Benazepril	Lotensin		
Quinapril	Accupril		
Moexipril	Univasc		
Fosinopril	Monopril		
Captopril	Capoten	9/10	
Trandolapril	Mavik		
Perindopril	Aceon		

DRUG CLASS: Angiotensin Receptor Blockers (ARBs)

DRUG NAMES, Generic	DRUG NAMES, Brand	NUTRIENTS DEPLETED	BW; Precautions; Populations
Losartan	Cozaar	5.5-10.5/3.5-7.5	**Fetal and neonatal morbidity and mortality.**
Olmesartan	Benicar	10-12/6-7	
Valsartan	Diovan	6-9/3-6	
Candesartan	Atacand	8-12/4-8	Malignancies, Renal Failure, Hyperkalemia. Less benefit in Black patients. No known nutrient depletions.
Irbesartan	Avapro	8-12/5-8	
Telmisartan	Micardis	6-13/6-8	
Azilsartan kamedoximil	Edarbi	12-14/6-9	

References: drugs.com (professional), https://www.rxlist.com/beta_blockers/drug-class.htm, https://www.straight-healthcare.com/alpha-2-agonists.html, https://my.clevelandclinic.org/health/treatments/22321-alpha-blockers Mitch Stargrove's "Herb, Nutrient and Drug Interactions"

APPENDIX A: Hypertension

Table 3: Nutrient Depletions and the secondary diagnoses they can cause.

DRUG CLASS	NUTRIENT WASTED	PROBLEMS CAUSED	FOOD SOURCES
Thiazide diuretics, Loop diuretics, Beta blockers	*CoQ-10*	Necessary cofactor in the mitochondria of cells to turn ADP into ATP—fatigue, physically and mentally (poor concentration, memory lapses, "negative" mood changes).	Meat, fish, nuts
Thiazide diuretics, Loop diuretics	*Magnesium*	Magnesium is distributed roughly 60% in bone, 25% in muscles, rest in soft tissues and fluids (gastric), so lack of this nutrient can look like fatigue, irritability, weakness, muscle tightness/spasms, dysmenorrhea, *hypertension*, cardiomyopathy, nerve conduction problems, anorexia, insomnia, sugar cravings, poor nail growth, anxiety.	Non-GMO soy flour/beans, buckwheat flour, whole wheat flour, rye flour, dried figs, black-eyed peas, Swiss chard, almonds, cashews, brown rice, kidney beans, hazelnuts, lima beans, baked halibut, Brazil nuts, kelp, peanuts, walnuts
Thiazide diuretics, Loop diuretics, ACE inhibitors	*Sodium (Na)*	Na/K: Altered acid-base balance, electrical activity for nerve/muscle cells altered, disrupted water balance and kidney/adrenal functioning	Sardines, flounder, haddock, peanut butter, salmon, cod, beef liver, artichoke, celery, tuna, leg of lamb, white turkey/chicken meat, pork
Thiazide diuretics, Loop diuretics, Calcium channel blocker (Amlodipine)	*Potassium (K)*	Muscle weakness, fatigue, mental confusion, irritability, arrhythmias, muscle cramps, abdominal bloating, nerve conduction abnormalities	Avocado, tomato sauce, dried apricots, potato, cantaloupe, papaya, prune juice, dried figs, lima beans, parsnips, cooked pumpkin, watermelon, raisins, kiwi, sardines

Diseases of the Drugs

DRUG CLASS	NUTRIENT WASTED	PROBLEMS CAUSED	FOOD SOURCES
Thiazide diuretics, Loop diuretics, Potassium-sparing diuretic (Triamterene), Calcium channel blocker (Amlodipine)	*Calcium*	Osteoporosis, osteomalacia, muscle spasms/tetany, *hypertension*, periodontal disease, hyperactivity, anxiety, insomnia	Cheeses, turnip greens, torula yeast, lambs quarters, sardines with bones, collard greens, rhubarb, dairy products, spinach, oatmeal
Thiazide diuretics, Loop diuretics, Potassium-sparing diuretic (Triamterene), ACE inhibitors	*Zinc*	Altered synthesis of cholesterol, protein, fats; dysregulation of release of vitamin A from liver; cell growth (epithelial tissue) adversely affected, prostate changes, vision changes, insulin dysregulation, immune system lessened, altered taste perception, loss of protection against heavy metal toxicity	Eastern oysters, Pacific oysters, roast beef, toasted wheat germ, dark turkey meat, cheeses, ground beef, lima beans, baked potato, rolled oats, mustard greens, pumpkin seeds
Thiazide diuretics, Calcium channel blocker (Amlodipine)	*Vitamin D*	Bone health compromised, Seasonal Affective Disorder, increased sensitivity to pain	Sunshine! Halibut liver oil, sardines, cod liver oil, mackerel, herring, tuna, salmon, shrimp
Loop diuretics	*Vitamin B1 (Thiamin)*	Mental confusion, disordered thinking, irritability, anorexia, muscle weakness & tenderness, indigestion, constipation, tachycardia, palpitations, edema, polyneuritis, difficulty walking, muscle wasting	Brewer's yeast, sunflower seeds, non-GMO soybeans, toasted wheat germ, beef kidney, navy beans, kidney beans, beef liver, dark rye flour, rolled oats, brown rice, whole wheat flour, chick peas, salmon steak, split peas

APPENDIX A: Hypertension

DRUG CLASS	NUTRIENT WASTED	PROBLEMS CAUSED	FOOD SOURCES
Loop diuretics	*Vitamin B6 (Pyridoxine)*	Depression, nausea/vomiting, mucous membrane lesions, seborrheic dermatitis, peripheral neuritis, ataxia, hyperacusis, hyperirritability, altered mobility & alertness, abnormal head movement, convulsions	Whole grain cereal (bran intact), broiled pork loin chop, watermelon, banana, salmon, avocado, light chicken/turkey meat without skin, beef liver, tomato juice, rainbow trout, steelhead trout, Atlantic mackerel, sunflower seeds
Loop diuretics	*Vitamin B12 (Cobalamin)*	Pernicious anemia, progressive peripheral neuropathy with pronounced anemia, fatigue, depression, confusion, memory loss, psychosis, glossitis, achlorhydria, impaired lymphocyte response, decreased phagocyte and PMN response, spinal degeneration, macrocytic cells	Much higher in animal sources than non-animal sources*: Beef liver, clams, salmon steak, lamb, lobster, beef, tuna, cheese; Also in brewer's yeast, nori, wakame, kombu, chlorella, spirulina. *Exception to the rule is "super blue green" algae.
Loop diuretics	*Vitamin C*	Listlessness, fatigue, weakness, shortness of breath, muscle cramps, aching bones/joints/muscles, anorexia, dry skin, fever, hemorrhage, easy bruising, secondary infections, corneal hypertrophy, swollen joints, bleeding gums	Acerola berries, orange juice, guava, peppers, grapefruit juice, watermelon, cantaloupe, honeydew, papaya, grapefruit, kiwi, Brussels sprouts, cauliflower, broccoli, mango, orange, turnip greens, strawberries
Loop diuretics, Potassium-sparing diuretic (Triamterene)	*Folic Acid (folate)*	Poor growth, megaloblastic anemia, glossitis, GI tract disturbances	Chicken liver, brewer's yeast, black-eyed peas, lentils, turnip greens, lima beans, orange juice, beef liver, kidney beans, peanuts, romaine lettuce, sprouted peas, dandelion greens

Diseases of the Drugs

DRUG CLASS	NUTRIENT WASTED	PROBLEMS CAUSED	FOOD SOURCES
Loop diuretics	*Mixed tocopherols (vitamin E)*	Dry skin, easy bruising, decreased clotting time, eczema, psoriasis, elevated heavy metals, PMS, cystic fibrosis, sickle cell anemia, beta thalassemia, cataracts, fibrocystic disease, BPH, poor wound healing, hot flashes, growing pains, Osgood-Schlatter disease	Wheat germ oil, sunflower seeds/oil, almonds/oil, pecans, hazelnuts, wild purslane, sweet potato, tempeh, safflower oil, flax oil, wheat germ
Loop diuretics	*Phosphorus*	Phosphorus is the second most abundant mineral in the body after calcium; 80% reside in calcium phosphate crystals in bone/teeth. A deficiency will adversely impact bones and teeth!	Cheeses, ham, dairy products; split pea soup, almonds, oatmeal, lentils
Beta blockers	*Melatonin*	dysregulation of sleep onset and quality, dysregulation of sex hormone production	Hormone is secreted by pineal gland, not available in food sources
Beta blockers	*Chromium*	glucose intolerance, elevated cholesterol & triglycerides	Calf liver, potato with skin, whole grain bread, green pepper, carrot, apple, cornmeal, brewer's yeast, banana, spinach, cabbage, orange, blueberries

APPENDIX A: Hypertension

Table 4: Commonly used excipients in anti-hypertensive agents

DRUG CLASS	EXCIPIENT	POTENTIAL PROBLEMS
Beta blockers	Acetyl tributyl citrate	A food additive with limited or no toxicity information available. Not suspected to be environmental toxin. Not expected to be potentially toxic or harmful. Not suspected to be persistent or bioaccumulative. **Restricted** per EWG.
Calcium channel blockers (part of shell)	Ammonium hydroxide	Caustic inorganic base. Persistent or bioaccumulative and moderate to high toxicity concerns in humans. Strong evidence of human toxicity or allergen. Expected to be toxic or harmful, especially if inhaled. Limited evidence of skin irritation. Wildlife and environmental toxin. Prohibited for use in food. Occupational handling hazard. **Restricted** per EWG.
Thiazide diuretics, Loops, Potassium sparers, Alpha agonists, Alpha blockers, Beta blockers, Calcium channel blockers, ACE inhibitors, ARBs	Anhydrous lactose or lactose monohydrate	Milk sugar may affect lactose-intolerant individuals.
Calcium channel blockers	Betadex	Limited or no toxicity information available, yet used in food or as additive. Uncertain environment toxicity, persistence, and bioaccumulation. Not expected to be potentially toxic or harmful, persistent, or bioaccumulative. **Restricted** per EWG.
ARBs	Calcium stearate	Calcium salt of stearic acid. Suspected to be environmental toxin. Risk assessment methods deficiencies and data gaps. Not expected to be potentially toxic or harmful. Not suspected to be persistent or bioaccumulative. **Restricted** per EWG.
ARBs	Carboxymethylcellulose calcium	Calcium salt of carboxymethylcellulose, commercially made from wood, chemically modified. GRAS.
Beta blockers	Carnauba wax	Extract from leaves of the Brazilian carnauba palm. Designated as "safe". Not suspected to be environmental toxin. Not expected to be potentially toxic or harmful.

DRUG CLASS	EXCIPIENT	POTENTIAL PROBLEMS
ACE inhibitors	Copovidone	Contamination concerns: vinyl acetate, 1-vinyl-2-pyrrolidone.
Loop diuretics, Potassium sparers, Alpha agonists, Alpha blockers, Beta blockers, Calcium channel blockers, ACE inhibitors, ARBs	Corn starch/maize starch	Not expected to be toxic or harmful. Author concern is for GMO/glyphosate contamination
Potassium sparers, Beta blockers, ACE inhibitors, ARBs	Croscarmellose sodium	Cross-linked polymer of cellulose gum. Limited data on safety.
Thiazide diuretics	Croscarmellose sodium-Type A	AVOID when eating the Specific Carbohydrate Diet; might cause harmful bacterial flora growth in the intestines. Derived from wood pulp and/or cotton fibers. https://healthfully.com/is-potassium-chloride-a-poison-6991454.html
Loops, Potassium sparers, Alpha blockers, Beta blockers, Calcium channel blockers, ACE inhibitors, ARBs	Crospovidone, polyvinyl-polypyrrolidone (PVP), povidone	Expected to be toxic or harmful. **Restricted** per EWG.
Alpha agonists, Calcium channel blockers (part of shell), ACE inhibitors (shell)	D&C Yellow #10	Synthetic dye produced from petroleum or coal tar. Contamination concerns: **zinc, aniline, cadmium.** Possible immune, allergenic, nervous system effects. Endocrine disruptor. Positive for mutations. Not expected to be bioaccumlative or environmental toxin. **Restricted-Unacceptable** per EWG.
Thiazides, Alpha blockers, Beta blockers, Calcium channel blockers (also on shell), ACE inhibitors	D&C Yellow #10 aluminum lake	Coal tar or petroleum-produced pigment adhered to aluminum; high concern of contamination with zinc, aniline, cadmium. Possible immune, allergenic, nervous system effects. Cancer concern. Associated with endocrine disruption. Suspected environmental toxin. **Restricted-Unacceptable** per EWG.

APPENDIX A: Hypertension

DRUG CLASS	EXCIPIENT	POTENTIAL PROBLEMS
ACE inhibitors	D&C Red #27 Aluminum Lake	Coal tar or petroleum produced pigment adhered to aluminum. Persistent or bioaccumulative and moderate to high toxicity concerns in humans. Persistent, bioaccumulative in wildlife. Wildlife and environmental toxicity. Expected to be toxic or harmful. Limited evidence of eye irritation. Associated with endocrine disruption. **Unacceptable** per EWG.
Thiazides	D&C Red #30 Aluminum Lake	Coal tar- or petroleum-produced pigment adhered to aluminum. Expected to be toxic/harmful. Suspected to be environmental toxin. Persistent, bioaccumulative in wildlife. Associated with endocrine disruption. **Unacceptable** per EWG.
Beta blockers, ACE inhibitors (shell)	D&C Red #28	Synthetic dye made from petroleum or coal tar. Persistent, bioaccumulative, moderate to high toxicity concerns in humans. Persistent, bioaccumulative in wildlife. Expected to be toxic or harmful. Associated with endocrine disruption. **Unacceptable** per EWG.
Potassium sparers, Alpha blockers, ACE inhibitors (shell)	D&C Red #33	Contamination concerns: biphenyl-2-ylamine. Otherwise, not considered toxic to humans or environment. **Unacceptable** per EWG.
Calcium channel blockers	Diethyl phthalate	Aromatic diester of ethyl alcohol and phthalic acid. Limited evidence of reproductive toxicity. Associated with endocrine disruption. Limited evidence of immune toxicity or allergies. Wildlife and environmental toxicity. Risk assessment deficiencies and data gaps. Not suspected to be bioaccumulative. **Unacceptable** per EWG.
Alpha agonists, Beta blockers, Calcium channel blockers	Ethyl cellulose	Ethyl ether of cellulose. Expected to be toxic or harmful to humans. Prohibited for use in food. **Restricted** per EWG.

DRUG CLASS	EXCIPIENT	POTENTIAL PROBLEMS
Calcium channel blockers	Ethyl acrylate copolymer	Ethyl acrylate is a reactive monomer that is highly irritating to the eyes, skin, mucous membranes, and may cause lethargy and seizures if concentrated vapor is inhaled. Found to be carcinogenic in rats in 1986, but delisted in 2000. Chemically combined with ethene, acrylic acid and its salts, amides and esters, methacrylates, acrylonitrile, maleic esters, vinyl acetate, vinyl chloride, vinylidene chloride, styrene, butadiene and unsaturated polyesters to form copolymers.
Thiazides, Alpha agonists, Alpha blockers, Beta blockers (inside and on shell), Calcium channel blockers, ACE inhibitors (shell)	FD&C Blue #1	Contamination concerns: aniline, cadmium. Neurotoxin. Endocrine disruptor. Moderate cancer concern. Produced from petroleum. Also used as textile dye and wood colorant. Triarylmethane dye. **Restricted-Unacceptable** status per EWG.
ACE inhibitors, Calcium channel blockers (shell)	FD&C Blue #1 aluminum lake	Typically synthetically produced from petroleum or coal tar. Precipitated to aluminum. Contamination concerns: aniline, cadmium. Banned or found unsafe in cosmetics. Persistent and bioaccumulative. Moderate to high toxicity concerns in humans. Classified as medium human health priority. Limited evidence of carcinogenicity. Used in food or as additive with limited to no toxicity information. Concern of neurotoxicity at any dose. Associated with endocrine disruption. **Restricted-Unacceptable** per EWG.
Alpha agonists, Beta blockers, ACE inhibitors (shell)	FD&C Blue #2	Banned in cosmetics. Tumor formation at moderate doses. Not considered bioaccumulative or environmental toxin.
Alpha blockers, Calcium channel blockers (also on shell), ACE inhibitors	FD&C Blue #2 Aluminum Lake	Tumor formation at moderate doses. Uncertain environmental toxin; uncertain bioaccumulation.

APPENDIX A: Hypertension

DRUG CLASS	EXCIPIENT	POTENTIAL PROBLEMS
Thiazides, Alpha blockers, Beta blockers (shell), Calcium channel blockers (shell)	FD&C Red #3	Persistence and bioaccumulation concern. Banned/found unsafe for use in cosmetics or around eyes, yet approved for prescription medications. **Unacceptable** status per EWG
Beta blockers, Calcium channel blockers (shell), ACE inhibitors (shell)	FD&C Red #40	Synthetic dye made from petroleum. Contamination concerns: mercury, aniline, cadmium, 6-methoxy-M-toluidine. Moderate evidence for human allergen or toxicant. Mutation evidence in mammals. Found to be persistent and bioaccumulative in wildlife. Associated with endocrine disruption. **Restricted** per EWG.
Thiazides, Alpha blockers, Calcium channel blockers (part of shell), ACE inhibitors	FD&C Red #40 aluminum lake	Coal tar- or petroleum-produced pigment adhered to aluminum; concern with contaminants: mercury, 6-methoxy-m-toluidine, aniline, cadmium. Possible human toxicant or allergen; possible neurotoxin; mutation results on mammalian cells; persistent and bioaccumulative in wildlife; endocrine disruptor. **Restricted** per EWG.
Potassium sparers, Beta blockers, Calcium channel blockers (part of shell), ACE inhibitors (shell)	FD&C Yellow #6	Contamination concerns: cadmium. Moderate evidence of human toxicant or allergen. Possibly toxic to reproduction or development. Weak endocrine disruption. Not expected to be bioaccumulative or an environmental toxin. **Restricted-Unacceptable** per EWG.
Calcium channel blockers (also in shell), ACE inhibitors	FD&C Yellow #6 Aluminum Lake	Petroleum or coal tar derivative precipitated to metal salt, typically aluminum (calcium, barium, or other). Contamination concern with cadmium. Moderate evidence of human toxicant or allergen. Possible neurotoxin and reproductive/developmental harm. Associated with endocrine disruption. **Restricted – Unacceptable** per EWG.
ARBs	Fumaric acid	A dicarboxylic acid classified as an irritant to eyes, skin, lungs. Risk assessment method deficiencies and data gaps. Not expected to be environment toxin. Not expected to potentially cause human harm. Not suspected to be persistent or bioaccumulative or carcinogenic in humans. **Restricted** per EWG.

DRUG CLASS	EXCIPIENT	POTENTIAL PROBLEMS
Thiazides, Potassium sparers, Alpha blockers (shell), Beta blockers (inside and part of shell), Calcium channel blockers (also part of shell), ACE inhibitors	Gelatin	Protein obtained from boiled animal connective tissue. Potentially toxic or harmful. **Restricted** per EWG
Calcium channel blockers (also part of shell), ARBs	Glycerin, glycerol	Naturally occurring alcohol compound, animal or vegetable origin. Restricted in cosmetics in Canada. Not expected to be potential health concern. **Restricted** per EWG.
Thiazides, Calcium channel blockers, ACE inhibitors	Glyceryl triacetate, triacetin	Expected to be toxic or harmful. **Restricted** per EWG.
Beta blockers	Hydrogenated vegetable oil	Usually hydrogenated soybean oil. Contains monosodium glutamate (MSG). Hydrogenation is process of adding hydrogen gas under high pressure to liquid oils. Used in making gas from coal and manufacturing margarine and shortening. This process of hydrogenation lead to *trans* fats. Risk assessment method deficiencies and data gaps.
Beta blockers	Hydroxyethyl cellulose	Modified cellulose polymer; thickening agent. Not suspected to be environmental toxin. Not expected to be potentially toxic or harmful. Data gaps. **Restricted** per EWG.
Calcium channel blockers, ARBs	Hydroxypropyl cellulose, low-substituted hydroxypropyl cellulose	Propylene glycol ether of cellulose. Risk assessment method deficiencies and data gaps. **Restricted** per EWG.

APPENDIX A: Hypertension

DRUG CLASS	EXCIPIENT	POTENTIAL PROBLEMS
Thiazides, Potassium sparers, Alpha agonists, Beta blockers, Calcium channel blockers, ACE inhibitors, ARBs	Hypromellose, hydroxypropyl methylcellulose	A semisynthetic polymer based on cellulose. **Restricted** per EWG.
Thiazides, Calcium channel blockers, ACE inhibitors, ARBs	Iron/ferric oxides: red, yellow, black	Persistent, bioaccumulative in wildlife and humans. Limited evidence of respiratory toxicity. Not suspected to be environmental toxin. Limited/incomplete evidence of cancer; data gaps. **Restricted** per EWG.
Calcium channel blockers (also part of shell)	Light mineral oil	Byproduct of petroleum industry. Eye irritant. Causes birth defects and cancer by inhalation. Strong evidence of respiratory toxicant or allergen. Expected to be toxic or harmful. **Restricted** per EWG.
ACE inhibitors	Magnesium carbonate	Prohibited for use in food. Not expected to be environmental toxin. Not expected to be potentially toxic or harmful.
Thiazides, Loops, Potassium sparers, Alpha agonists, Alpha blockers, Beta blockers, Calcium channel blockers, ACE inhibitors, ARBs	Magnesium stearate	Data gaps and risk assessment method deficiencies. Uncertain environmental toxin, uncertain persistent or bioaccumulative. **Restricted** per EWG.
ARBs	Mannitol	A hexahydric alcohol. Not suspected to be an environmental toxin. Not expected to be potentially toxic or harmful. Not suspected to be persistent or bioaccumulative. **Restricted** per EWG.
ARBs	Meglumine, methylglucamine	A form of sorbitol, a sugar alcohol. Often used in conjunction with iodinated organic compounds as a contrast medium. Not suspected to be an environmental toxin, persistent nor bioaccumulative. Not expected to be potentially toxic or harmful.

Diseases of the Drugs

DRUG CLASS	EXCIPIENT	POTENTIAL PROBLEMS
Calcium channel blockers	Methacrylic acid	Use is restricted in Canadian cosmetics. Allowed workplace exposures restricted to low doses. Occupational hazards related to handling. Classified as toxic or harmful. **Unacceptable** per EWG.
Calcium channel blockers (part of shell)	Methyl paraben	Parabens mimic estrogen. Associated with endocrine disruption. Interferes with gene expression. Moderate evidence of human immune toxicant or allergen. Risk assessment method deficiencies and data gaps. Not suspected to be persistent or bioaccumulative. Not expected to be potentially toxic or harmful. Not suspected to be environmental toxin. Methyl paraben is **Restricted** per EWG.
Beta blockers	Methylene chloride, dichloromethane	Known human respiratory toxicant. Limited evidence of gastric or liver toxicity. Banned or found unsafe for use in cosmetics. Possible human carcinogen. Persistent, bioaccumulative in wildlife. Limited evidence of reproductive toxicity. Wildlife and environmental toxicity. **Unacceptable** per EWG.
Thiazides, Loops, Potassium sparers, Alpha agonists, Alpha blockers, Beta blockers, Calcium channel blockers, ACE inhibitors, ARBs	Microcrystalline cellulose	Strong evidence of human immune and respiratory toxicant or allergen.
Potassium sparers	Opadry yellow	Hypromellose, titanium dioxide, **macrogol,** iron oxide yellow, polysorbate 80, and iron oxide red
ARBs	Opadry white	OPADRY is a "complete film coating system" and trademarked product of Colorcon. Opadry—the original, customized, one-step film coating system combining polymer, plasticizer, and pigment in a dry concentrate." Allows for "sharp logo definition." Contains lactose monohydrate, Hypromellose, titanium dioxide, and PEG/macrogol

APPENDIX A: Hypertension

DRUG CLASS	EXCIPIENT	POTENTIAL PROBLEMS
Calcium channel blockers (part of shell)	Propyl paraben	Parabens mimic estrogen. Strong evidence of endocrine disruption. Significant wildlife and environmental disruption. Strong evidence of human immune toxicant or allergen. Possible human reproductive or developmental toxin. Risk assessment method deficiencies and data gaps. **Unacceptable** per EWG.
Thiazides, Calcium channel blockers, ACE inhibitors	Polydextrose	Limited data. Random polymer formed from condensation of D-glucose.
Thiazides, Alpha agonists, Beta blockers, Calcium channel blockers, ACE inhibitors, ARBs	Polyethylene glycol	Petroleum derivative. Growing concern of anaphylaxis. https://pubmed.ncbi.nlm.nih.gov/33011299/
Beta blockers, Calcium channel blockers	Polysorbate	Contamination concerns: ethylene oxide, 1-4 dioxane. Limited evidence of sense organ toxicity. Not expected to be environmental toxin.
Potassium sparers, Alpha agonists, Beta blockers	Polysorbate 80, Sorbitan	Contamination concerns: ethylene dioxide, a known human carcinogen, unsafe for use in cosmetics, known respiratory toxicant, limited evidence of kidney toxicity, eye/lung/skin irritant, strong evidence of human immune toxicant; not expected to be bioaccumulative or environmental toxin. **Unacceptable** per EWG); and 1,4-dioxane, a synthetic industrial material, completely miscible in water, unstable at higher temperatures/pressure, explosive with prolonged exposure to light/air, resistant to biodegradation, likely to be carcinogenic, upper respiratory, kidney and liver damage. https://www.epa.gov/sites/default/files/2014-03/documents/ffrro_factsheet_contaminant_14-dioxane_january2014_final.pdf
ACE inhibitors	Polyvinyl alcohol	Risk assessment method deficiencies and data gaps. Limited or incomplete evidence of cancer (data gaps). **Restricted** per EWG.

DRUG CLASS	EXCIPIENT	POTENTIAL PROBLEMS
Thiazides, Loops, Alpha agonists, Beta blockers (and maize and partially pregelatinized), Calcium channel blockers, ACE inhibitors, ARBs	Pregelatinized starch	Vegan/vegetarian "gelatin." Contamination concern: pesticides. Risk assessment method deficiencies and data gaps. **Restricted** per EWG.
Calcium channel blockers	Saccharin sodium	Artificial sweetener. Used in food or as additive with limited or no toxicity information available. Limited or incomplete evidence of cancer. Controversial over the years.
Thiazides, Loops, Potassium sparers, Alpha blockers, Beta blocker, Calcium channel blockers (inside and on shell)	Sodium lauryl sulfate	Topical irritant. Expected to be toxic or harmful. Suspected to be an environmental toxin. Risk assessment method deficiencies and data gaps. **Restricted** per EWG.
Thiazides, Loops, Potassium sparers, Beta blockers, Calcium channel blockers	Sodium starch glycolate	Sodium salt of carboxymethyl ether from rice, potato, wheat, or corn. Medium human health priority. **Restricted** per EWG.
Thiazides	Sodium Starch glycolate type-A	Something new on the market approved by the WHO in 2020. May be sourced from potato, corn, or "unspecified ingredient". https://precision.fda.gov/ginas/app/ui/substances/H8AV0SQX4D
ARBs	Sodium hydroxide	"Caustic soda", a highly caustic and reactive inorganic base. Expected to be toxic or harmful. Medium human health priority. Occupational hazards related to handling. Not suspected to be bioaccumulative. **Restricted** per EWG.
Beta blockers, ACE inhibitors	Sodium stearyl fumarate	Causes skin irritation. Causes serious eye irritation. (PubChem)

APPENDIX A: Hypertension

DRUG CLASS	EXCIPIENT	POTENTIAL PROBLEMS
Calcium channel blockers (part of shell)	Sorbitol	Sugar alcohol. Not suspected to be environmental toxin. Not expected to be potentially harmful or toxic. Not suspected to be persistent or bioaccumulative. **Restricted** per EWG.
Alpha agonists, Beta blockers, ACE inhibitors	Stearic acid	Naturally occurring fatty acid, usually obtained from rendered fat of domestic and farm animals. Suspected to be environmental toxin. Not likely to be carcinogenic. Not expected to be harmful or toxic. Not suspected to be persistent or bioaccumulative.
Alpha blockers, Beta blockers	Sucrose	"Table sugar." Not suspected to be environmental toxin. Not expected to be toxic or harmful. Not suspected to be persistent or bioaccumulative.
Beta blockers, Calcium channel blockers	Sugar spheres	Sugar + starch, layered (for timed-release products)
Thiazides, Potassium sparers, Alpha blockers, Beta blockers, ACE inhibitors	Talc	Native/natural. Sometimes contains aluminum silicate. Can be contaminated with asbestos. Asbestos-free, cosmetic-grade talc is a form of magnesium silicate shown to be toxic and carcinogenic. NOT known to be an environmental toxin, persistent or bioaccumulative. **Restricted to Unacceptable** per EWG.
Thiazides, Potassium sparers, Alpha blockers (shell), Beta blockers (inside and on shell), Calcium channel blockers (inside and on shell), ACE inhibitors, ARBs	Titanium dioxide	White pigment from minerals. Possible human carcinogen. Expected to be toxic or harmful. **Restricted** per EWG.
ACE inhibitors	Zinc stearate	Zinc salt of stearic acid. Persistent or bioaccumulative and moderate to high toxicity concerns in humans. Persistent, bioaccumulative in wildlife. Expected to be toxic or harmful. Suspected to be environmental toxin.

DRUG CLASS	EXCIPIENT	POTENTIAL PROBLEMS
What's *on* that capsule?	Black ink containing…	
Thiazides, ACE inhibitors	Black iron oxide	Persistent, bioaccumulative in wildlife and humans. Limited evidence of respiratory toxicity. Not suspected to be environmental toxin. Limited/incomplete evidence of cancer; data gaps. **Restricted** per EWG.
Thiazides, Alpha blockers, Calcium channel blockers, ACE inhibitors	Butyl alcohol, n-butyl alcohol	Known human lung and skin toxicant. Expected to be toxic or harmful. Data gaps. **Restricted** per EWG.
Thiazides	Dehydrated alcohol	"Absolute" alcohol: not less than 99.2% alcohol by weight or 99.5% by volume. Sclerosing agent.
Thiazides	Isopropyl alcohol	First commercial synthetic alcohol. Reaction of propylene (petroleum by-product) with sulfuric acid, then hydrolysis. US Government has regulations in place for the amount of isopropyl alcohol allowed in foods.
Loops, Potassium sparers, Alpha blockers (inside shell), Beta blockers, Calcium channel blockers	Potassium hydroxide	Classified as toxic or harmful. Wildlife and environmental toxicity concern. **Restricted** per EWG.
Thiazides, Alpha blockers, Calcium channel blockers, ACE inhibitors	Propylene glycol (trimethyl glycol, methyl ethyl glycol, dihydroxypropane, propanediol)	Skin irritant; penetration enhancer. Expected to be toxic or harmful. Various grades used in foods, engine coolants, airplane deicing, antifreeze, enamels, paints. About 45% eliminated via kidneys; rest turned into lactic acid. Potential interaction with metformin and lactic acid toxicity! https://www.webmd.com/diet/what-to-know-about-propylene-glycol-in-foods
Calcium channel blockers	SD-45 alcohol	Specially denatured alcohol. Grain-derived, considered broadly toxic. Penetration enhancer. Persistent, bioaccumulative in wildlife. Used in food or as additive with little to no toxicity information available. Limited evidence of sense organ, gastrointestinal, or liver toxicity. Limited evidence of cancer. Occupational hazards related to handling. Unknown risk to nervous system.

APPENDIX A: Hypertension

DRUG CLASS	EXCIPIENT	POTENTIAL PROBLEMS
Thiazides, Alpha blockers, Beta blockers, Calcium channel blockers, ACE inhibitors	Shellac	Resin secreted by lac bug in Thailand and India. Used as colorant, food glaze, wood finish. Natural glue.
Thiazides, Alpha blockers, Beta blockers, Calcium channel blockers	Strong ammonia solution	Amidase inhibitor and neurotoxin. Manufactured and produced naturally by bacterial processes and breakdown of organic matter.

www.Drugs.com/pro; A Consumer's Dictionary of Food Additives, Ruth Winter, MS; www.ewg.org; Opadry white (https://pharm.unideb.hu/sites/default/files/upload_documents/8._analytical-procedures.pdf) and https://www.colorcon.com/markets/pharmaceuticals

What about "gelatin"—from what is that derived? Great question, Reader! Mostly, gelatin comes from animal bones, cartilage and skin. *Dare I ask what animals are used for their bones, cartilage and skin?* Cows, chickens, pigs and fish, most commonly.

ROLLING BLOOD PRESSURE NUMBERS

DATE	Range of week	Before breakfast	Mid-morning	Random (note time)	Mid-afternoon	After supper	Random (note time)	Before bedtime
	SUNDAY	MONDAY	TUESDAY	WEDNESDAY	THURSDAY	FRIDAY	SATURDAY	

APPENDIX B
Dyslipidemia

Table 1: Drugs that can cause dyslipidemia

Table 2: Drugs used to manage dyslipidemia, warnings/precautions, efficacy, nutrients wasted

Table 3: Nutrient deficiencies caused by the drugs used to manage dyslipidemia, food sources

Table 4: Other ingredients in drugs used to manage dyslipidemia

Table 1

Listed below are some of the drugs that can increase the risk of being diagnosed with high total cholesterol, LDL, and/or triglycerides:

Thiazide diuretics

Drug name, generic	Drug name, brand	Indications for use
Chlorothiazide Hydrochlorothiazide Chlorthalidone Metolazone	Diuril HydroDiuril Hygroton, Thalitone Zaroxolyn	Fluid accumulation; sometimes high blood pressure

Loop diuretics

Drug name, generic	Drug name, brand	Indications for use
Furosemide Torsemide	Lasix Demadex	Fluid accumulation, high blood pressure

Beta blockers

Drug name, generic	Drug name, brand	Indications for use
Metoprolol Betaxolol Bisoprolol Timolol Carvedilol	Toprol, Lopressor Kerlone Zebeta Timoptic, Blocadren Coreg	High blood pressure; some also have approved indications for use in heart failure, migraine prevention, to prevent a second heart attack, chest pain

"Mood stabilizers"

Drug name, generic	Drug name, brand	Indications for use
Lithium	Eskalith, Lithobid	Bipolar disorder (patients age 7 and older)

APPENDIX B: Dyslipidemia

Anti-psychotics (often used as "mood stabilizers")

Drug name, generic	Drug name, brand	Indications for use
Aripiprazole Risperidone Olanzapine Ziprasidone Quetiapine Lurasidone Clozapine	Abilify Risperdal, Perseris Zyprexa Geodon Seroquel Latuda Clozaril, FasaClo, Versacloz	Schizophrenia; sometimes approved for use in major depressive disorder, bipolar disorder, suicidal behavior in schizophrenia or schizoaffective disorder, irritability in autism, bipolar mania, Tourette's disorder

Anti-convulsants (often used as "mood stabilizers")

Drug name, generic	Drug name, brand	Indications for use
Gabapentin Phenytoin Lamotrigine Divalproex	Neurontin, Gralise Dilantin Lamictal Depakote	Partial (focal) seizures; others are indicated for use in nerve pain after shingles, generalized seizures, status epilepticus, bipolar disorder, mania, migraines,

Steroids

Drug name, generic	Drug name, brand	Indications for use
Prednisone Betamethasone Cortisone Hydrocortisone Dexamethasone Clobetasol Methylprednisolone Prednisolone Triamcinolone Desonide Desoximetasone	Deltasone Diprolene Compound E Cortef, Solu-Cortef Decadron Clobex, Temovate Medrol Oropred, Millipred Kenalog Desowen, Tridesilon Topicort	Anti-inflammatory or immune suppressant agents across most body systems and conditions: allergic, neoplastic, skin, blood, gut, eyes, joints, skin, immune, nervous, endocrine, respiratory, kidney; solid organ rejection. Used by mouth, applied to the skin, inhaled into the nose or mouth, or injected.

Hormones (progestins)

Drug name, generic	Drug name, brand	Indications for use
Medroxyprogesterone Levonorgestrel (found in IUD, mini-pills & combo oral contraceptives, too)	Provera, Depo-Provera Mirena, Lyletta, Skyla, Kyleena; Plan B, Next Choice, My Way, React, Option 2, Aftera	Contraception and heavy menstrual bleeding; medroxyprogesterone is also indicated for use in lack of menstrual bleeding, endometriosis, endometrial overgrowth and cancer.

Hormones (estrogens)

Drug name, generic	Drug name, brand	Indications for use
Estrone	Kestrone-5, Estragyn/LA 5, EstroneAQ, Aquest	Peri/post-menopausal symptoms, various cancers, bHRT, atrophic urethritis and vaginitis, dyspareunia, primary ovarian failure, HRT, contraception, abnormal uterine bleeding, gender dysphoria
Estradiol	Estrace, Estradiol Patch, Climara, Vagifem, Estring, Imvexxy	
Estriol	Ovestin, Evelon, Femastin, Gynest	
Ethinyl estradiol		
Conjugated estrogens	Premarin, Cenestin, Enjuvia	
Estropipate	Ogen, Ortho-Est	
Diethylstilbestrol	Stilphostrol	

Hormones (androgens)

Drug name, generic	Drug name, brand	Indications for use
Fluoxymesterone Methyltestosterone Oxymetholone	Halotesten, Androxy Methitest, Testred Anadrol-50	Primary hypogonadism, hypogonadotropic hypogonadism, certain cancers, delayed puberty; anemia

APPENDIX B: Dyslipidemia

Anti-depressants, tricyclics, SNRI, SSRIs

Drug name, generic	Drug name, brand	Indications for use
Amitriptyline Desipramine Doxepin Imipramine Notriptyline Venlafaxine Paroxetine Citalopram Escitalopram Fluoxetine Sertraline	Elavil Norpramin Sinequan, Silenor Tofranil Pamelor Effexor Paxil Celexa Lexapro Prozac Zoloft	Major depressive disorder; some have indications for use in bipolar disorder, sleep issues, anxiety, bed-wetting https://healthfully.com/zoloft-and-cholesterol-6020923.html https://pubmed.ncbi.nlm.nih.gov/23798963/

Retinoids

Drug name, generic	Drug name, brand	Indications for use
Isotretinoin Tazarotene* Tretinoin^ Acetretin* (incr/decr cholesterol; incr TG) Bexarotene+	Absorica, Accutane, Claravis, Myorisan, Sotret, Zenatane Arazlo, Avage, Fabior, Tazorac Vesanoid, Retin-A, Altreno, Stieva-A Soriatane Targretin	Acne, aesthetics; plaque psoriasis*; acute promyelocytic leukemia, necrobiosis lipoidica diabeticorum, photoaging of skin, and lichen sclerosis^; skin lesions caused by cutaneous T-cell lymphoma+ https://www.singlecare.com/drug-classes/retinoids

Bile acid sequestrants

Drug name, generic	Drug name, brand	Indications for use
Cholestyramine+ Colestipol^+ Colesevelam *	Questran, Prevalite Colestid Welchol	Used to bind dietary cholesterol in the gut lumen to lower total cholesterol

Anti-retrovirals; protease inhibitors

Drug name, generic	Drug name, brand	Indications for use
Tipranavir	Aptivus	Used in AIDS and HIV treatment
Atazanavir	Reyataz	https://www.verywellhealth.com/
Atazanavir/cobicistat	Evotaz	which-drugs-can-raise-cholesterol-levels-
Lopinavir/ritonavir	Kaletra	698229#toc-protease-inhibitors
Fosamprenavir	Lexiva	
Ritonavir	Norvir	
Darunavir	Prezista	
Darunavir/cobicistat	Prezcobix	

Monoclonal antibodies

Drug name, generic	Drug name, brand	Indications for use
Adalimumab	Humira	Autoimmune disorders, including certain
Pembrolizumab	Keytruda	cancers; osteoporosis (denosumab/Prolia)
Certolizumab	Cimzia	
Golimumab	Simponi	
Infliximab	Remicade	
Tocilizumab	Actemra	https://www.thehealthsite.com/
Basiliximab	Simulect	diseases-conditions/is-your-medication-raising-
Denosumab	Prolia	your-cholesterol-f0218-556867/

Lifestyle choices

Drug name, generic	Drug name, brand	Indications for use
Alcohol		
Cigarette smoking		

Table 2

Below are the drugs currently used to *treat* cholesterol abnormalities. The average drop in total cholesterol (TC) is also listed. (Optimal triglycerides: 70-110mg/dl, total cholesterol: 15-220mg/dl, LDL: <120mg/dl, HDL: 55-90mg.dl.) *All should be used in conjunction with lifestyle changes!*

Bile acid sequestrants

DRUG NAMES, Generic	DRUG NAMES, Brand	AVG DROP in TC	WARNINGS; Nutrients wasted
Cholestyramine+	Questran, Prevalite	LDL: 15-30%	Deficiencies in fat-soluble vitamins, constipation
Colesevelam *	Colestid	Can INCREASE TG and CAUSE acute pancreatitis	*GI obstruction, contains phenylalanine
Colestipol^+	Welchol		^GI obstruction, chest pain
			+Cancer
			Omega-3 fatty acids
			Beta-carotenes
			Calcium
			Folate
			Iron
			Zinc
			Vitamins:
			B2, 3, 12
			A, D, E, K

Fibrates

DRUG NAMES, Generic	DRUG NAMES, Brand	AVG DROP in TC	WARNINGS; Nutrients wasted
*Clofibrate	Atromid-S	Can cause decreases in HDL-C	Hepatotoxicity, myopathy, rhabdomyolysis, cholelithiasis, pancreatitis, hematological changes, venothrombotic diseases.
Gemfibrozil	Lopid		
Fenofibrate	Tricor, Antera, Triglide, Lofibra, Lipofen, Fenoglide		*Vitamin E*
			Zinc
			Copper(?)
Fenofibric acid	Trilipix, Fibricor		*CoQ-10(?)*
			Raise homocysteine,
			(B12, B6, folate)

Absorption inhibitor

DRUG NAMES, Generic	DRUG NAMES, Brand	AVG DROP in TC	WARNINGS; Nutrients wasted
Ezetimibe	Zetia	TC: -12 LDL-C: -18 ApoB: -16 TG: -8 HDL: +1	Upper respiratory tract infections, hepatitis, pancreatitis, cholecystitis, cholelithiasis. No known nutrient depletions

Statins

DRUG NAMES, Generic	DRUG NAMES, Brand	AVG DROP in TC	WARNINGS; Nutrients wasted
Atorvastatin	Lipitor	(27, 36, 30, 18, +7)	**Pregnancy category X! Contraindicated in pregnancy!** **Can cause birth defects and/or fetal death.** Myopathy, rhabdomyolysis, immune-mediated necrotizing myopathy, liver dysfunction, endocrine dysfunction, CNS toxicity. *CoQ-10 depletion.*
Fluvastatin	Lescol	(19, 14, 25, 18, +4)	
Lovastatin	Altoprev, Mevacor	(19, 27, 20, 6, +7)	
Pitavastatin	Livalo	(36, 30, 26, 19, +7)	
Pravastatin	Pravachol	(17, 23, 17, 9, +8)	
Rosuvastatin	Crestor	(34, 31, -, 37, +22)	
Simvastatin	Zocor	(24, 30, 30, 15, +7)	
		Class action suit against maker of atorvastatin for causing type 2 diabetes.	

Miscellaneous antihyperlipidemic agent

DRUG NAMES, Generic	DRUG NAMES, Brand	AVG DROP in TC	WARNINGS; Nutrients wasted
Bempedoic acid	Nexletol	Used as an add-on with maximum dose tolerated statin	Hyperuricemia (gout), tendon rupture

APPENDIX B: Dyslipidemia

PCSK9 inhibitors

DRUG NAMES, Generic	DRUG NAMES, Brand	AVG DROP in TC	WARNINGS; Nutrients wasted
Alirocumab Evolocumab	Praluent Repatha	(36, 58, 50, -, -) (36, 63, 49, -, -)	Watch for hypersensitivity reactions and immune system dysfunction (systemic illness, even sepsis)

Natural agent

DRUG NAMES, Generic	DRUG NAMES, Brand	AVG DROP in TC	WARNINGS; Nutrients wasted
Niacin/nicotinic acid	SloNiacin, Niacor, Niaspan	(8, 12, 12, 13, -)	Do *not* use concomitantly with statins.

Combinations

DRUG NAMES, Generic	DRUG NAMES, Brand	AVG DROP in TC	WARNINGS; Nutrients wasted
Simvastatin + ezetimibe Atorvastatin + amlodipine	Vytorin Caduet		**Pregnancy category X! Contraindicated in pregnancy! Can cause birth defects and/or fetal death.**

https://www.verywellhealth.com/what-are-bile-acid-sequestrants-697489

*Clofibrate patented in 1958 by Imperial Chemical Industries, approved for medical use in 1963, discontinued in 2002 d/t adverse events: SIADH, gallstones, death. Clofibrate - Wikipedia About 30% excess deaths: malignancy, cholecystectomy complications, pancreatitis; cousins' profiles are similar, but not as stark.

https://www.citizen.org/article/petition-to-require-a-box-warning-on-all-statins/ 2014. Request rejected. Cerivastatin pulled from market 2001 d/t rhabdomyolysis and deaths.

Table 3 Cholesterol Nutrient Deficiencies

DRUGS CLASS	NUTRIENT WASTED	PROBLEMS CAUSED	FOOD SOURCES
Bile acid sequestrants	Omega-3 fatty acids (require Zn, Mg, vitamins C, B6, B3, E, biotin, B5)	Increased clotting, increased inflammation, increased cell permeability, increased triglycerides, decreased HDL	Flax seed, hemp, canola, walnut, pumpkin, soy, algae, green plants, purslane, wild-caught cold-water fish
Bile acid sequestrants	Beta-carotenes (converted to vitamin A in the intestinal mucosa, primarily; rely on dietary fats and bile salts for absorption) [Carotenoids are precursors of vitamin A, which is active in 3 forms (retinol/alcohol, retinal/aldehyde, and retinoic acid/acid); beta-carotene has 2 retinal molecules, yet only 1/3 are absorbed. For these reasons, they're in the same box.] Vitamin A (requires protein, zinc for release from liver)	Vision loss/night blindness, dry eyes, macular degeneration; respiratory infections, follicular hyperkeratosis, reduced immunity, diarrhea, loss of tooth enamel, loss of bone mass, loss of taste and smell.	Dunaliella salina, carrot juice, spirulina, dandelion leaf, cod liver oil, burdock, sweet potato, carrot, mango, cooked pumpkin (think "orange" and "greens"!) Polar bear liver, beef liver, chicken liver, pork liver

APPENDIX B: Dyslipidemia

DRUGS CLASS	NUTRIENT WASTED	PROBLEMS CAUSED	FOOD SOURCES
Bile acid sequestrants	Calcium	Osteoporosis, osteomalacia, muscle spasms/tetany, hypertension, periodontal disease, hyperactivity, anxiety, insomnia	Cheeses, turnip greens, torula yeast, lambs quarters, sardines with bones, collard greens, rhubarb, dairy products, spinach, oatmeal
Bile acid sequestrants Fibrates, Niacin (both raise homocysteine)	Folate	Poor growth, megaloblastic anemia, glossitis, GI tract disturbances	Chicken liver, brewer's yeast, black-eyed peas, lentils, turnip greens, lima beans, orange juice, beef liver, kidney beans, peanuts, romaine lettuce, sprouted peas, dandelion greens
Bile acid sequestrants	Iron	Anemia, glossitis, nail spooning, increased susceptibility to infection, brittle nails, canker sores, hair loss, decreased endurance, impaired mental ability.	Beef liver, tofu, blackstrap molasses, cooked amaranth, oysters, cooked lentils, Swiss chard, ground beef, roast beef, dried dulse, lima beans, baked potato, mustard greens
Bile acid sequestrants Fibrates	Zinc	Altered synthesis of cholesterol, protein, fats; dysregulation of release of vitamin A from liver; cell growth (epithelial tissue) adversely affected, prostate changes, vision changes, insulin dysregulation, immune system lessened, altered taste perception, loss of protection against heavy metal toxicity	Eastern oysters, Pacific oysters, roast beef, toasted wheat germ, dark turkey meat, cheeses, ground beef, lima beans, baked potato, rolled oats, mustard greens, pumpkin seeds
Bile acid sequestrants	Vitamin B2 (Riboflavin)	Usually occurs in concert with other B vitamin deficiencies (seen here); cheilosis, glossitis, dry/scaly skin, itchy eyes, light sensitivity.	Beef kidney and liver, chicken liver, calf and beef heart, yogurt, cooked broccoli, almonds, brewer's yeast, cheeses (brie, Camembert, Roquefort, skim ricotta, Swiss), raw wild rice, dried soybeans

DRUGS CLASS	NUTRIENT WASTED	PROBLEMS CAUSED	FOOD SOURCES
Bile acid sequestrants	Vitamin B3 (Niacin)	Dermatitis (exacerbated by sun exposure), diarrhea, dementia, death!	Beef liver, canned (water-packed) tuna, light chicken meat, beef kidney, swordfish, salmon, halibut, peanuts, lean beef, chicken liver, cod, brown rice, sunflower seeds, almonds, whole wheat flour, dried soybeans, egg
Bile acid sequestrants Fibrates, Niacin (both raise homocysteine)	Vitamin B12	Pernicious anemia, progressive peripheral neuropathy with pronounced anemia, fatigue, depression, confusion, memory loss, psychosis, glossitis, achlorhydria, impaired lymphocyte response, decreased phagocyte and PMN response, spinal degeneration, macrocytic cells	Much higher in animal sources than non-animal sources*: Beef liver, clams, salmon steak, lamb, lobster, beef, tuna, cheese; brewer's yeast, nori, wakame, kombu, chlorella, spirulina *"Super blue-green" algae* is the exception to the rule,
Bile acid sequestrants	Vitamin D	Rickets in children, osteomalacia in adults—malformation or skeletal demineralization of bones. Increased sensitivity to pain. Seasonal Affective Disorder (SAD).	Halibut liver oil, sardines, cod liver oil, mackerel, herring, tuna, salmon, shrimp, mushrooms (morel, shitake, chanterelle), pork, halibut, egg yolk, lamb, beef
Bile acid sequestrants Fibrates	Vitamin E	Dry skin, easy bruising, decreased clotting time, eczema, psoriasis, elevated heavy metals, PMS, cystic fibrosis, sickle cell anemia, beta thalassemia, cataracts, fibrocystic disease, BPH, poor wound healing, hot flashes, growing pains, Osgood-Schlatter disease	Wheat germ oil, sunflower seeds/oil, almonds/oil, pecans, hazelnuts, wild purslane, sweet potato, tempeh, safflower oil, flax oil, wheat germ

APPENDIX B: Dyslipidemia

DRUGS CLASS	NUTRIENT WASTED	PROBLEMS CAUSED	FOOD SOURCES
Bile acid sequestrants	Vitamin K	Hemorrhagic disease of the newborn, spontaneous nosebleeds in children, osteoporosis	Turnip greens, cooked broccoli, cooked cabbage, beef liver, green tea, lettuce, raw spinach, asparagus, cooked oats, cheese, watercress, peach, peas, green beans, milk
Fibrates (possibly)	Copper	Breakdown of RBC (liver/brain damage), anemia, neutropenia, degeneration of vasculature, depigmentation of skin, kinky hair, hypotonia, hypothermia. Essential for moving iron from liver.	Beef liver, rye, dried beans, Brazil nuts, cashews, dried peas, blackstrap molasses, sunflower seeds, raw mushrooms, firm tofu, refried beans, almonds, whole wheat flour
Statins, Fibrates (possibly)	CoQ-10	Fatigue, diminished energy (inside the cell, as well as how the individual feels), cellular damage	Meats, fish, seeds
Fibrates, Niacin (both raise homocysteine)	B6	Depression, nausea, vomiting, mucous membrane lesions, seborrheic dermatitis, peripheral neuritis; ataxia, hyperacusis, hyperirritability, altered mobility and alertness, abnormal head movements, convulsions.	100% bran cereal, 40% bran cereal, broiled pork loin chop, watermelon, banana, raw salmon, avocado, light chicken meat (no skin), light turkey meat (no skin), beef liver, tomato juice, raw rainbow trout, raw steelhead salmon, raw Atlantic mackerel, sunflower seeds
Absorption inhibitor (ezetimibe) Misc. antihyperlipidemic agent (bempedoic acid) PCSK9 inhibitors	None known These are too new on the market to know just yet.		

Table 4 Excipients in the Dyslipidemic Managers

Excipients	Potential problems
Ascorbic acid	Vitamin C, sort of. Linus Pauling warned us about this.
Black iron oxide	Persistent, bioaccumulative in wildlife and humans. Limited evidence of respiratory toxicity.
Butylated hydroxyanisole	Petroleum-derived preservative. Banned in Japan. Suspected human carcinogen.
Calcium carbonate	Chalk. Occurs naturally in limestone, marble, coral.
Calcium stearate	Calcium salt of stearic acid. Suspected to be environmental toxin.
Cellacefate	Polymer phthalate. A concerning and controversial plastic.
Copovidone	Contamination concerns: vinyl acetate, 1-vinyl-2-pyrrolidone.
Croscarmellose sodium	Cross-linked polymer of cellulose gum. Limited data.
Crospovidone	Expected to be toxic or harmful.
D&C Yellow No. 10 aluminum lake	Coal tar- or petroleum-produced pigment adhered to aluminum; high concern with contaminants: zinc, aniline, cadmium. Possible immune, allergenic, nervous system effects. Cancer concern. Associated with endocrine disruption. Suspected environmental toxin.
Diacetylated monoglycerides	Glycerin esterified with edible fat-forming fatty acids and acetic acid. May be prepared with triacetin (below).
FD&C Blue #1 aluminum lake	Typically synthetically produced from petroleum or coal tar. Precipitated to aluminum. Contamination concerns: aniline, cadmium. Banned or found unsafe in cosmetics. Persistent and bioaccumulative with moderate to high toxicity concerns in humans. Classified as medium human health priority. Limited evidence of carcinogenicity. Used in food or as additive with limited to no toxicity information. Concern of neurotoxicity at any dose. Associated with endocrine disruption.
FD&C Blue #2 aluminum lake	Tumor formation at moderate doses. Uncertain environmental toxin; uncertain bioaccumulation.
FD&C Yellow #6 aluminum lake	Petroleum or coal tar derivative precipitated to metal salt, typically aluminum (calcium, barium or other). Contamination concern with cadmium. Moderate evidence of human toxicant or allergen. Possible neurotoxin and reproductive/developmental harm. Associated with endocrine disruption.
Ferrosoferric oxide	Black magnetic iron oxide.
Gelatin	Protein obtained from boiled animal connective tissue. Potentially toxic or harmful.

APPENDIX B: Dyslipidemia

Excipients	Potential problems
Hydroxypropyl cellulose	Propylene glycol ether of cellulose.
Hypromellose	A semisynthetic polymer based on cellulose.
Hypromellose 2910	Cellulose-based polymer. "Natural tears"
Lactose anhydrous, monohydrate	Milk sugar, potential problem for lactose-intolerant people.
Magnesium stearate	Data gaps and risk assessment method deficiencies. Uncertain environmental toxin, uncertain persistent or bioaccumulative. **Restricted** per EWG.
Maltodextrin	High glycemic index starch-based sweetener.
Medium-chain triglycerides	Obtained from palm tree oil and coconut oil, then esterified into new triglycerides.
Methacrylic acid - ethyl acrylate copolymer (1:1) type A	Methacrylic acid: Use is restricted in Canadian cosmetics. Allowed workplace exposures restricted to low doses. Occupational hazards related to handling. Classified as toxic or harmful. **Unacceptable** per EWG.
Methylcellulose	Thickener, emulsifier, bulk-forming laxative. Often main ingredient of wallpaper paste.
Microcrystalline cellulose	Strong evidence of human immune and respiratory toxicant or allergen.
Opadry white	Contains lactose monohydrate, hypromellose, titanium dioxide, PEG/macrogol.
Polydextrose	Reduced-calorie bulking agent by Pfizer.
Polyethylene glycol	Petroleum derivative. Growing concern of anaphylaxis. https://pubmed.ncbi.nlm.nih.gov/33011299/
Polysorbate 80	Contamination concerns: ethylene dioxide—a known human carcinogen, unsafe for use in cosmetics, known respiratory toxicant, limited evidence of kidney toxicity, eye/lung/skin irritant, strong evidence of human immune toxicant; not expected to be bioaccumulative or environmental toxin. **Unacceptable** per EWG—and 1,4-dioxane (synthetic industrial material, completely miscible in water, unstable at higher temperatures/pressure, explosive with prolonged exposure to light/air, resistant to biodegradation, likely to be carcinogenic, upper respiratory, kidney and liver damage.) https://www.epa.gov/sites/default/files/2014-03/documents/ffrro_factsheet_contaminant_14-dioxane_january2014_final.pdf
Povidone K30	Polyvinylpyrrolidone. Synthetic polymer, binder, suspending agent.

Excipients	Potential problems
Pregelatinized corn starch	Not expected to be toxic or harmful. Author concern is for GMO/glyphosate contamination. Vegan/vegetarian "gelatin." Contamination concern: pesticides.
Propylene glycol alginate	Propylene glycol ester of alginic acid derived from seaweed. Can cause allergic reactions.
Red iron oxide	Persistent, bioaccumulative in wildlife and humans. Limited evidence of respiratory toxicity.
Simethicone emulsion (30%)	Anti-flatulence remedy.
Sodium carbonate anhydrous	Soda ash. Neutralizer, processing agent. Strong alkali.
Sodium lauryl sulphate	Topical irritant. Expected to be toxic or harmful. Suspected to be an environmental toxin.
Sodium starch glycolate	Sodium salt of carboxymethyl ether from rice, potato, wheat or corn. Medium human health priority.
Sodium stearyl fumarate	Causes skin irritation. Causes serious eye irritation. (PubChem)
Sucrose (429.5 mg/g in cholestyramine!)	Table sugar.
Talc	Native/natural. Sometimes contains aluminum silicate. Can be contaminated with asbestos. Asbestos-free, cosmetic-grade talc is a form of magnesium silicate shown to be toxic and carcinogenic.
Titanium dioxide	White pigment from minerals. Possible human carcinogen. Expected to be toxic or harmful.
Triacetin	Expected to be toxic or harmful.
Triethyl citrate	Citric acid.
Yellow iron oxide	Persistent, bioaccumulative in wildlife and humans. Limited evidence of respiratory toxicity.
External Shell	
Ammonium hydroxide	Caustic inorganic base. Persistent or bioaccumulative and moderate to high toxicity concerns in humans. Strong evidence of human toxicity or allergen. Expected to be toxic or harmful (more so if/when inhaled). Limited evidence of skin irritation. Wildlife and environmental toxin. Prohibited for use in food. Occupational handling hazard.
Black iron oxide	Persistent, bioaccumulative in wildlife and humans. Limited evidence of respiratory toxicity.

APPENDIX B: Dyslipidemia

Excipients	Potential problems
Partially hydrolyzed polyvinyl alcohol	Risk assessment method deficiencies and data gaps. Limited or incomplete evidence of cancer (data gaps). **Restricted** per EWG.
Polyethylene glycol	Petroleum derivative. Growing concern of anaphylaxis. https://pubmed.ncbi.nlm.nih.gov/33011299/
Potassium hydroxide	Classified as toxic or harmful. Wildlife and environmental toxicity concern.
Propylene glycol	Skin irritant; penetration enhancer. Expected to be toxic or harmful. Various grades used in foods, engine coolants, airplane deicing, antifreeze, enamels, paints. About 45% eliminated via kidneys; rest turned into lactic acid. Potential interaction with metformin and lactic acid toxicity! https://www.webmd.com/diet/what-to-know-about-propylene-glycol-in-foods
Shellac	Resin secreted by lac bug in Thailand and India. Used as colorant, food glaze, wood finish. Natural glue.
Talc	Native/natural. Sometimes contains aluminum silicate. Can be contaminated with asbestos. Asbestos-free, cosmetic-grade talc is a form of magnesium silicate shown to be toxic and carcinogenic.
Titanium dioxide	White pigment from minerals. Possible human carcinogen. Expected to be toxic or harmful.
Injectables	
Histidine	Essential amino acid.
Polysorbate 20	Derived from lauric acid (palm kernel, coconut oils). Contamination concerns (ethylene glycols, ethylene oxide).
Sucrose (100 mg, alirocumab)	Table sugar.
Polysorbate 80	Contamination concerns: ethylene dioxide (known human carcinogen, unsafe for use in cosmetics, known respiratory toxicant, limited evidence of kidney toxicity, eye/lung/skin irritant, strong evidence of human immune toxicant; not expected to be bioaccumulative or environmental toxin. **Unacceptable** per EWG), and 1,4-dioxane (synthetic industrial material, completely miscible in water, unstable at higher temperatures/pressure, explosive with prolonged exposure to light/air, resistant to biodegradation, likely to be carcinogenic, upper respiratory, kidney and liver damage.) https://www.epa.gov/sites/default/files/2014-03/documents/ffrro_factsheet_contaminant_14-dioxane_january2014_final.pdf
Proline (25-89 mg, evolocumab)	Non-essential amino acid.

www.Drugs.com/pro; A Consumer's Dictionary of Food Additives, Ruth Winter, MS; www.ewg.org

APPENDIX C
Type 2 Diabetes

Table 1: Drugs that can cause type 2 diabetes

Table 2: Drugs used to manage type 2 diabetes, warnings/precautions, efficacy, nutrients wasted.

Table 3: Nutrient deficiencies caused by the drugs used to manage type 2 diabetes, food sources

Table 4: Other ingredients in drugs used to manage type 2 diabetes

Rolling Blood Glucose Log

Table 1

Below are some of the drugs that can increase the risk of being diagnosed with type 2 diabetes:

Drug name, generic	Drug name, brand	Drug class	Indications for use
Chlorothiazide Hydrochlorothiazide Chlorthalidone Metolazone	Diuril HydroDiuril Hygroton, Thalitone Zaroxolyn	Thiazide diuretics	Fluid accumulation; sometimes high blood pressure
Furosemide Torsemide	Lasix Demadex	Loop diuretics	Fluid accumulation, high blood pressure
Metoprolol Betaxolol Bisoprolol Timolol Carvedilol	Toprol, Lopressor Kerlone Zebeta Timoptic, Blocadren Coreg	Beta blockers	High blood pressure; some also have approved indications for use in heart failure, chest pain, migraine prevention, to prevent a second heart attack
Albuterol Levalbuterol	Ventolin, Proventil, ProAir Xopenex	Short acting beta-2 agonists; bronchodilators	Bronchospasm; albuterol has indication for exercise-induced bronchospasm
Formoterol (+budesonide) Salmeterol (+fluticasone)	Forodil, Perforomist (Symbicort) Serevent (Advair, AirDuo)	Long acting beta-2 agonists; bronchodilators	Asthma, COPD (emphysema, chronic bronchitis), exercise-induced bronchospasm
Theophylline	TheoDur, Theocron, Theo-24, Elixophyllin	Methylxanthine; bronchodilator	Asthma, COPD
Atorvastatin Simvastatin Rosuvastatin Fluvastatin Pitavastatin	Lipitor FloLipid, Zocor Crestor, Ezallor Lescol Levalo	"Statins" Anti-lipemic agents (lipid lowering agents)	High cholesterol levels (adults and children), to reduce the risk of heart attack, stroke, chest pain, stent placement in patients with/without past history of any of the above who also have multiple coronary heart disease risk factors; some are also approved for high triglycerides & special types of lipid irregularities

APPENDIX C: Type 2 Diabetes

Drug name, generic	Drug name, brand	Drug class	Indications for use
Niacin	Slo-Niacin, Niacor, Niaspan	Vit. B3; Lowers lipids	Various kinds of lipid abnormalities
Lithium	Eskalith, Lithobid	Anti-mania	Bipolar disorder (7+ years)
Aripiprazole Risperidone Olanzapine Ziprasidone Quetiapine Lurasidone Clozapine	Abilify Risperdal, Perseris Zyprexa Geodon Seroquel Latuda Clozaril	Anti-psychotics, often called "mood stabilizers"	Schizophrenia; some also have approval for use in major depressive disorder, bipolar disorder, suicidal behavior in schizophrenia or schizoaffective disorder, bipolar mania, Tourette's
Gabapentin Phenytoin Lamotrigine Divalproex	Neurontin, Gralise Dilantin Lamictal Depakote	Anti-convulsants or anti-epileptics, often called "mood stabilizers"	Partial (focal) seizures; others are indicated for nerve pain after shingles, generalized seizures, status epilepticus, bipolar disorder, mania, migraines,
Prednisone Betamethasone Cortisone Hydrocortisone Dexamethasone Clobetasol Methylprednisolone Prednisolone Triamcinolone Desonide Desoximetasone	Deltasone Diprolene Compound E Cortef, Solu-Cortef Decadron Clobex, Temovate Medrol Oropred, Millipred Kenalog Desowen, Tridesilon Topicort	Corticosteroids	Anti-inflammatory or immune suppressant agents across most body systems and conditions: allergic, neoplastic, skin, blood, gut, eyes, joints, skin, immune, nervous, endocrine, respiratory, kidney; solid organ rejection. Used by mouth, applied to the skin, inhaled into the nose or mouth, or injected.
Medroxyprogesterone Levonorgestrel (found in mini-pills & combo contraceptives, too)	Provera, Depo-Provera Mirena, Lyletta, Skyla, Kyleena; Plan B, Next Choice, My Way, React, Option 2, Aftera	Progestins	Contraception and heavy menstrual bleeding; medroxyprogesterone is also indicated for use in lack of menstrual bleeding, endometriosis, endometrial overgrowth and cancer.
Febuxostat	Uloric	Xanthine deriv.	Gout

Diseases of the Drugs

Drug name, generic	Drug name, brand	Drug class	Indications for use
Modafinil	Provigil	Central nervous system stimulant	Narcolepsy, obstructive sleep apnea, shift work sleep disorder
Amitriptyline Desipramine Doxepin Imipramine Notriptyline Bupropion*	Elavil Norpramin Sinequan, Silenor Tofranil Pamelor Wellbutrin/XL, Zyban	Tricyclic anti-depressants Atypical/NDRI anti-depressant	Major depressive disorder; some have indications for use in bipolar disorder, sleep issues, anxiety, bed-wetting; smoking cessation* (hypo or hyperglycemia)
Moxifloxacin Ciprofloxacin Levofloxacin	Avelox Cipro Levaquin	Antibiotics, fluoroquinolones	All kinds of infections that are *susceptible* to these agents. Can cause HYPOglycemia!
Clonidine Epinephrine	Catapres/Kapvay Primatene Mist	Alpha-2 agonist Non-specific	Hypertension/ADD/ADHD Asthma (OTC product)
Bevacizumab Ipilimumab Pembrolizumab Rituximab Golimumab Basiliximab	Avastin Yervoy Keytruda Rituxan Simponi Simulect	Monoclonal antibodies can cause **type 1** diabetes as well as **type 2**!	Used in autoimmune conditions including cancers.
Isotretinoin Acetretin^ Bexarotene+	Absorica, Accutane Soriatane Targretin	Retinoids ^incr/decr gluc.	Acne, aesthetics; skin lesions caused by cutaneous T-cell lymphoma+
Tipranavir (Atazanavir)/cobicistat Lopinavir/(ritonavir) Fosamprenavir (Darunavir)/cobicistat	Aptivus (Reyataz) Evotaz Kaletra (Norvir) Lexiva (Prezista) Prezcobix	Anti-retrovirals, protease inhibitors	Used in the treatment of HIV and AIDS

Table 2

Below are the drugs currently used to *treat* type 2 diabetes. The average drop in hemoglobin A1c (HbA1c) is also listed. HbA1c is roughly an average blood glucose over the past 2-3 months. **Every drug listed is to be used "as an adjunct to diet and exercise"**. (Normal HbA1c is 4.0-5.6%, pre-diabetes is 5.7-6.4%, diabetes is 6.5% and higher.)

Sulfonylureas

DRUG NAMES, Generic	DRUG NAMES, Brand	AVG DROP in HbA1c	BOXED WARNING; *Nutrients wasted*
Glyburide Glipizide Glimepiride	Diabeta, Glycron, Glynase, Micronase Glucotrol Amaryl	1-2%	CoQ10 *Magnesium* (diabetics tend to be deficient in Mg before drug therapy) Hypoglycemia

Biguanides

DRUG NAMES, Generic	DRUG NAMES, Brand	AVG DROP in HbA1c	BOXED WARNING; *Nutrients wasted*
Metformin	Glucophage	1-2%	**Lactic acidosis** Diarrhea *Folic acid* *Vitamin B12*

α-glucosidase inhibitors

DRUG NAMES, Generic	DRUG NAMES, Brand	AVG DROP in HbA1c	BOXED WARNING; *Nutrients wasted*
Acarbose Miglitol	Precose Glyset	0.5%	Abdominal pain, diarrhea, flatulence. Post-marketing: rare fulminant hepatitis, pneumatosis cystoides intestinalis.

Thiazolidinediones (aka "glitazones")

DRUG NAMES, Generic	DRUG NAMES, Brand	AVG DROP in HbA1c	BOXED WARNING; *Nutrients wasted*
Rosiglitazone Pioglitazone	Avandia Actos	1-1.5%	**Congestive heart failure;** bladder cancer, hepatic failure, edema, bone fractures, macular edema.

Meglitinides (aka "glinides")

DRUG NAMES, Generic	DRUG NAMES, Brand	AVG DROP in HbA1c	BOXED WARNING; *Nutrients wasted*
Repaglinide Nateglinide	Prandin Starlix	1-1.5% Do not pair with NPH insulin	Hypoglycemia

Glucagon-like Peptide receptor-1 (GLP-1) agonists

DRUG NAMES, Generic	DRUG NAMES, Brand	AVG DROP in HbA1c	BOXED WARNING; *Nutrients wasted*
*Exenatide (synthetic) Lixisenatide (synthetic) *Dulaglutide (grown on Chinese hamster ovary cells) *Liraglutide (grown on Saccharomyces cerevisiae) *Semaglutide (grown on Saccharomyces cerevisiae)	Bydureon, Byetta Adlyxin Trulicity Victoza Ozempic	1% Do not pair with insulin or sulfonylureas (hypoglycemia)	***Thyroid C-cell tumors and medullary thyroid cancer;** acute pancreatitis, acute kidney injury, severe GI disease (class action suit), immunogenicity (antibody production), thrombocytopenia, gallbladder disease, diabetic retinopathy, hypoglycemia, pulmonary aspiration during deep sedation or anesthesia

Amylin analog

DRUG NAMES, Generic	DRUG NAMES, Brand	AVG DROP in HbA1c	BOXED WARNING; *Nutrients wasted*
Pramlintide (synthetic)	Symlin	0.4-0.6%	**Severe hypoglycemia** (list of patient criteria prior to prescribing)

DiPeptidyl Peptase-4 (DPP-4) inhibitors

DRUG NAMES, Generic	DRUG NAMES, Brand	AVG DROP in HbA1c	BOXED WARNING; *Nutrients wasted*
Sitagliptin Saxagliptin Linagliptin	Januvia Onglyza Tradjenta	0.8% Do not pair with insulin or sulfonylureas (hypoglycemia)	Pancreatitis, heart failure, acute renal failure, severe arthralgias, bullous pemphigoid.

Sodium-Glucose co-transporter Type-2 (SGLT-2) inhibitors

DRUG NAMES, Generic	DRUG NAMES, Brand	AVG DROP in HbA1c	BOXED WARNING; *Nutrients wasted*
*Canagliflozin Empagliflozin^ Dapagliflozin	Inkovana Jardiance Farxiga	0.6-1.2% Do not pair with insulin or sulfonylureas (hypoglycemia)	*Limb amputations (dropped to mere Warning/Precaution in Aug 2020), volume depletion/hypotension, ketoacidosis, urosepsis, pyelonephritis, necrotizing fasciitis, genital mycotic infections, bone fractures, kidney injury, incr LDL-C^

Table 3

Nutrients wasted by medications used to manage type 2 diabetes and food sources to replenish.

DRUG CLASS	NUTRIENT WASTED	PROBLEMS CAUSED	FOOD SOURCES
Sulfonylureas	Coenzyme Q-10	Necessary cofactor in the mitochondria of cells to turn ADP into ATP—fatigue, physically and mentally (poor concentration, memory lapses, "negative" mood changes).	Meat, fish, nuts.
Sulfonylureas	Magnesium	Magnesium levels affect bones (60%), muscles (25%) soft tissues, and digestive fluids. Deficiency can cause fatigue, irritability, weakness, muscle tightness/spasms, dysmenorrhea, *hypertension*, cardiomyopathy, nerve conduction problems, anorexia, insomnia, sugar cravings, poor nail growth, anxiety.	Non-GMO soy flour/beans, buckwheat flour, whole wheat flour, rye flour, dried figs, black-eyed peas, Swiss chard, almonds, cashews, brown rice, kidney beans, hazelnuts, lima beans, baked halibut, Brazil nuts, kelp, peanuts, walnuts
Biguanide (metformin)	Folate	Poor growth, megaloblastic anemia, glossitis, GI tract disturbances	Chicken liver, brewer's yeast, black-eyed peas, lentils, turnip greens, lima beans, orange juice, beef liver, kidney beans, peanuts, romaine lettuce, sprouted peas, dandelion greens
Biguanide (metformin)	B12	Pernicious anemia, progressive peripheral neuropathy with pronounced anemia, fatigue, depression, confusion, memory loss, psychosis, glossitis, achlorhydria, impaired lymphocyte response, decreased phagocyte and PMN response, spinal degeneration, macrocytic cells	Much higher in animal sources than non-animal sources*: Beef liver, clams, salmon steak, lamb, lobster, beef, tuna, cheese; brewer's yeast, nori, wakame, kombu, chlorella, spirulina. *"Super blue green" algae is the exception to the rule.

Table 4

Excipients used in type 2 diabetes medications

EXCIPIENTS	PROBLEMS
Copovidone	Contamination concerns: vinyl acetate, 1-vinyl-2-pyrrolidone.
Corn starch	Not expected to be toxic or harmful. Author concern is for GMO/glyphosate contamination
Croscarmellose sodium	Cross-linked polymer of cellulose gum. Limited data.
D&C yellow # 10 aluminium lake	Coal tar or petroleum produced pigment adhered to aluminum; high concern with contaminants: zinc, aniline, cadmium. Possible immune, allergenic, nervous system effects. Cancer concern. Associated with endocrine disruption. Suspected environmental toxin.
FD&C blue #1/ brilliant blue FCF aluminium lake	Typically synthetically produced from petroleum or coal tar. Precipitated to aluminum. Contamination concerns: aniline, cadmium. Banned or found unsafe in cosmetics. Persistent of bioaccumulative and moderate to high toxicity concerns in humans. Classified as medium human health priority. Limited evidence of carcinogenicity. Used in food or as additive with limited to no toxicity information. Concern of neurotoxicity at any dose. Associated with endocrine disruption.
FD&C Blue No.1	Contamination concerns: aniline, cadmium. Neurotoxin. Endocrine disruptor. Moderate cancer concern. Produced from petroleum. Textile dye, wood stain, colorant. Triarylmethane dye.
FD&C Red No.40	Synthetic dye made from petroleum. Contamination concerns: mercury, aniline, cadmium, 6-methoxy-M-toluidine. Moderate evidence for human allergen or toxicant. Mutation evidence in mammals. Found to be persistent and bioaccumulative in wildlife. Associated with endocrine disruption. **Restricted** per EWG.
FD&C Yellow #6/ Sunset Yellow Aluminum Lake	Petroleum or coal tar derivative precipitated to metal salt, typically aluminum (calcium, barium or other). Contamination concern with cadmium. Moderate evidence of human toxicant or allergen. Possible neurotoxin and reproductive/developmental harm. Associated with endocrine disruption. **Restricted – Unacceptable** per EWG.
Ferric oxide red/ yellow	Persistent, bioaccumulative in wildlife and humans. Limited evidence of respiratory toxicity. Not suspected to be environmental toxin. Limited/incomplete evidence of cancer; data gaps. **Restricted** per EWG.
Hydrochloric acid	Strong acid. (Our own stomachs make this! For pharmaceuticals, it's made in a lab.)

EXCIPIENTS	PROBLEMS
Hydroxypropyl cellulose	Propylene glycol ether of cellulose. Risk assessment method deficiencies and data gaps. **Restricted** per EWG.
Lactose monohydrate	What about the lactose-intolerant?
Magnesium stearate	Data gaps and risk assessment method deficiencies. Uncertain environmental toxin, uncertain persistent or bioaccumulative. **Restricted** per EWG.
Magnesium stearate (E572)	Vegetable-sourced
Malic acid	In food, flavoring agent; in cosmetics, exfoliating agent. Only the L-form occurs in nature.
Mannitol	A hexahydric alcohol. Not suspected to be an environmental toxin. Not expected to be potentially toxic or harmful. Not suspected to be persistent or bioaccumulative. **Restricted** per EWG.
Microcrystalline cellulose	Strong evidence of human immune and respiratory toxicant or allergen.
Polacrilin potassium	Polacrilin potassium is an ion exchange resin used in oral pharmaceutical formulations as a tablet disintegrant. It is a weakly acidic cation exchange resin. Chemically, it is a partial potassium salt of a copolymer of methacrylic acid with divinyl benzene. Physically, ion exchange resins are small plastic beads with a diameter of roughly 0.6 millimeters. https://www.drugs.com/inactive/polacrilin-potassium-39.html
Poloxamer 188	Wound cleaner; under investigation for use in chronic microvascular diseases. https://go.drugbank.com/drugs/DB11333
Polyethylene glycol	Petroleum derivative. Growing concern of anaphylaxis. https://pubmed.ncbi.nlm.nih.gov/33011299/
Polyethylene glycol 3000	Solvent, carrier, modifying agent.
Polysorbate 80	Contamination concerns: ethylene dioxide (known human carcinogen, unsafe for use in cosmetics, known respiratory toxicant, limited evidence of kidney toxicity, eye/lung/skin irritant, strong evidence of human immune toxicant; not expected to be bioaccumulative or environmental toxin. **Unacceptable** per EWG), 1,4-dioxane (synthetic industrial material, completely miscible in water, unstable at higher temperatures/pressure, explosive with prolonged exposure to light/air, resistant to biodegradation, likely to be carcinogenic, upper respiratory, kidney and liver damage.) https://www.epa.gov/sites/default/files/2014-03/documents/ffrro_factsheet_contaminant_14-dioxane_january2014_final.pdf

APPENDIX C: Type 2 Diabetes

EXCIPIENTS	PROBLEMS
Polyvinyl alcohol	Risk assessment method deficiencies and data gaps. Limited or incomplete evidence of cancer (data gaps). **Restricted** per EWG.
Povidone, K-30, K-90	Polyvinylpyrrolidone. Synthetic polymer, binder, suspending agent
Pregelatinized starch	Vegan/vegetarian "gelatin" Contamination concern: pesticides. Risk assessment method deficiencies and data gaps. **Restricted** per EWG.
Pregelatinized maize starch	Used for ease of fast-manufacturing.
Sodium hydroxide	Highly caustic and reactive inorganic base. "Caustic soda." Expected to be toxic or harmful. Medium human health priority. Occupational hazards related to handling. Not suspected to be bioaccumulative. **Restricted** per EWG.
Sodium starch glycolate	Sodium salt of carboxymethyl ether from rice, potato, wheat or corn. Medium human health priority. **Restricted** per EWG.
Synthetic red/yellow iron oxide	Made in a lab rather than harvested from natural iron
Talc	Native/natural. Sometimes contains aluminum silicate. Can be contaminated with asbestos. Asbestos-free, cosmetic-grade talc is a form of magnesium silicate shown to be toxic and carcinogenic. Not known to be an environmental toxin, persistent or bioaccumulative. **Restricted to Unacceptable** per EWG.
Titanium dioxide	White pigment from minerals. Possible human carcinogen. Expected to be toxic or harmful. **Restricted** per EWG.
Triacetin	Expected to be toxic or harmful. **Restricted** per EWG.
Yellow iron oxide	Persistent, bioaccumulative in wildlife and humans. Limited evidence of respiratory toxicity. Not suspected to be environmental toxin. Limited/incomplete evidence of cancer; data gaps. **Restricted** per EWG.
EXTERNAL SHELL	
Ammonium hydroxide	Caustic inorganic base. Persistent or bioaccumulative and moderate to high toxicity concerns in humans. Strong evidence of human toxicity or allergen. Expected to be toxic or harmful (more so if/when inhaled). Limited evidence of skin irritation. Wildlife and environmental toxin. Prohibited for use in food. Occupational handling hazard.
Artificial blackberry flavor	Synthetic compound designed to mimic the taste of blackberries.

EXCIPIENTS	PROBLEMS
Black iron oxide	Persistent, bioaccumulative in wildlife and humans. Limited evidence of respiratory toxicity. Not suspected to be environmental toxin. Limited/incomplete evidence of cancer; data gaps. **Restricted** per EWG.
FD&C Yellow #6 Aluminum Lake	Petroleum or coal tar derivative precipitated to metal salt, typically aluminum (calcium, barium or other). Contamination concern with cadmium. Moderate evidence of human toxicant or allergen. Possible neurotoxin and reproductive/developmental harm. Associated with endocrine disruption. **Restricted – Unacceptable** per EWG.
Ferrosoferric oxide	Black magnetic iron oxide.
Hypromellose	A semisynthetic polymer based on cellulose.
Iron oxide yellow	Persistent, bioaccumulative in wildlife and humans. Limited evidence of respiratory toxicity. Not suspected to be environmental toxin. Limited/incomplete evidence of cancer; data gaps. **Restricted** per EWG.
Polyethylene glycol/macrogol	Petroleum derivative. Growing concern of anaphylaxis. https://pubmed.ncbi.nlm.nih.gov/33011299/
Polyvinyl alcohol	Water-soluble synthetic polymer.
Red ferric oxide	Persistent, bioaccumulative in wildlife and humans. Limited evidence of respiratory toxicity. Not suspected to be environmental toxin. Limited/incomplete evidence of cancer; data gaps. **Restricted** per EWG.
Shellac glaze	Glaze made from resin secreted by lac bug in Thailand and India. Used as colorant, food glaze, wood finish. Natural glue.
Talc	Native/natural. Sometimes contains aluminum silicate. Can be contaminated with asbestos. Asbestos-free, cosmetic-grade talc is a form of magnesium silicate shown to be toxic and carcinogenic. NOT known to be an environmental toxin, persistent or bioaccumulative. **Restricted to Unacceptable** per EWG.
Titanium dioxide	White pigment from minerals. Possible human carcinogen. Expected to be toxic or harmful. **Restricted** per EWG.
INJECTIONS	
Acetic acid	Buffering agent
Citric acid anhydrous	Not expected to be harmful to humans or environment
Disodium phosphate dihydrate, 1.42 mg	Emulsifier, preservative, pH modifying agent.
D-mannitol	Tonicity modifier; a hexahydric alcohol. Not suspected to be an environmental toxin. Not expected to be potentially toxic or harmful. Not suspected to be persistent or bioaccumulative. **Restricted** per EWG.

APPENDIX C: Type 2 Diabetes

EXCIPIENTS	PROBLEMS
Glacial acetic acid	Buffering solution
Glycerol 85% (54 mg)	The "backbone" of lipids known as glycerides. Food sweetener; pharmaceutical humectant.
Hydrochloric acid	Buffering agent
Mannitol (23.2 mg)	Tonicity-adjusting agent. A hexahydric alcohol. Not suspected to be an environmental toxin. Not expected to be potentially toxic or harmful. Not suspected to be persistent or bioaccumulative. **Restricted** per EWG.
Metacresol (2.2mg-8.1mg)	Antimicrobial preservative
Methionine (9.0 mg)	Amino acid
Phenol, 5.5 mg	Obtained from coal tar, used in manufacturing. Ingestion of small amounts may cause nausea, vomiting, circulatory collapse, paralysis, convulsions, coma, respiratory failure, cardiac arrest. Antiseptic, general disinfectant.
Polysorbate 80 (0.10-0.125mg)	Contamination concerns: ethylene dioxide (known human carcinogen, unsafe for use in cosmetics, known respiratory toxicant, limited evidence of kidney toxicity, eye/lung/skin irritant, strong evidence of human immune toxicant; not expected to be bioaccumulative or environmental toxin. **Unacceptable** per EWG), 1,4-dioxane (synthetic industrial material, completely miscible in water, unstable at higher temperatures/pressure, explosive with prolonged exposure to light/air, resistant to biodegradation, likely to be carcinogenic, upper respiratory, kidney and liver damage.) https://www.epa.gov/sites/default/files/2014-03/documents/ffrro_factsheet_contaminant_14-dioxane_january2014_final.pdf
Propylene glycol, 14 mg	Defoaming additive, emulsifier, antifreeze in breweries and dairy establishments.
Sodium acetate (trihydrate)	Buffering agent
Sodium hydroxide	Buffering agent. Highly caustic and reactive inorganic base. "Caustic soda". Expected to be toxic or harmful. Medium human health priority. Occupational hazards related to handling. Not suspected to be bioaccumulative. **Restricted** per EWG.
Trisodium citrate dihydrate (1.37 mg)	Antioxidant, emulsifier, sequestrant, stabilizer.
Water for injections	

www.Drugs.com/pro; A Consumer's Dictionary of Food Additives, Ruth Winter, MS; www.ewg.org

ROLLING BLOOD GLUCOSE NUMBERS

	Before breakfast	Mid-morning	Random (note time)	Mid-afternoon	After supper	Random (note time)	Before bedtime
SUNDAY							
MONDAY							
TUESDAY							
WEDNESDAY							
THURSDAY							
FRIDAY							
SATURDAY							

DISEASE REVERSAL

Vol. 1: Cardiometabolic Issues

Christie Fleetwood, ND, RPh, FNMI, cBC

Table of Contents

Building a strong foundation	4
Creating your map	12
Top 10 myths and stumbling blocks	14
Naturopathic medicine's history/philosophy	17
Physical body: food, water, movement, sleep	22
Food	22
Skin food	29
Advanced topics in food	30
Drink clean water	33
Advanced topics in water	36
Move your body	37
Get radically restorative sleep	38
Delving into…Emotions-Mind-Spirit	39
Live life on purpose	39
Make relationships healthy	39
Non-edible consumptions	42
Have you lost yourself	43
How to talk to prescribers about deprescribing	47
About A.M.	49
Final remarks to followers of YHWH	51
References and Resources	59
Naturopathic Basics	61

Disease Reversal: Hypertension, Dyslipidemia, Type 2 Diabetes

WARNING: DO NOT TAKE YOURSELF OFF YOUR PRESCRIPTION MEDICATION!

De-prescribing needs to be a team effort! Keep track of your subjective symptoms and objective signs (information on that is coming up). Watch for over-medication, then show your documentation to your prescriber with the request to reduce or remove medication.

ANY DEVIATION FROM THIS SEQUENCE CAN PUT YOU AT RISK!

I absolutely want to educate you, and I absolutely hope you choose disease reversal instead of chronic disease management. I trust that you are diligently tracking your progress, because above all else, I desire to keep you safe.

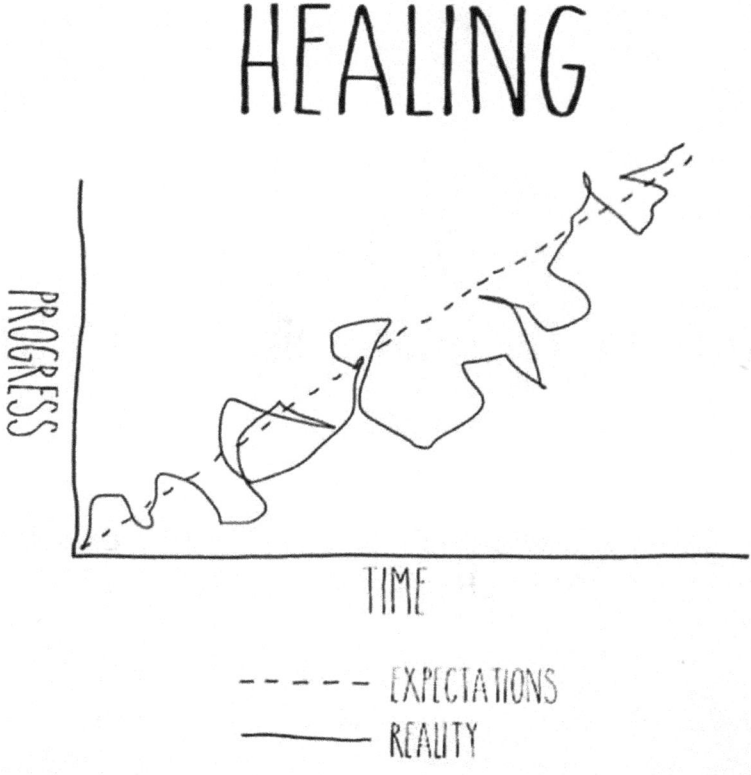

Graph by Josh Pogonitz

Congratulations! How absolutely fabulous to find you here!

- You've made it through the first half of this book which, I'm told, is *depressing*. *"It's such a downer, Doc!"* Um, it's called "Diseases of the Drugs." It's really not meant to be uplifting. It **is** meant to give you *informed consent* with subsequent *medical choice*. Which leads us to bullet point number two…
- You've decided you're at least interested in knowing what disease reversal entails. Awesome! I *adore* informed, curious-for-more readers!
- You are a fraction of the population. Go, YOU, for being the unique individual that you are! So many people choose disease management over taking control of their own health and lives.

A pharmacy customer once thanked me for being more interested in his health than he was. He liked his current lifestyle and wasn't interested in changing it the least bit, even though he could only afford to buy his prescription pills a few at a time.

My first naturopathic office was housed inside a compounding pharmacy; one of their regular pharmacy customers called frequently, begging for help. It was quite dramatic and disturbing. She was routed to me and I set up an appointment for us to meet. On the phone, she told me she had chronic fatigue (CF), fibromyalgia (FM) and irritable bowel syndrome (IBS) so badly she couldn't eat anything. She cried and pleaded for help, saying she was always in pain all over her body.

Disease Reversal: Hypertension, Dyslipidemia, Type 2 Diabetes

She arrived with her husband, both of them probably in their late sixties. He was in a nice suit and she was wearing lovely jewelry. For someone who couldn't eat anything, she was much larger than I'd expected. The three of us squeezed into my tiny office space—basically a repurposed closet with just enough room for a treatment table and a little chair in the corner. Since the door opened inward, hitting against the table, we had to enter single file with him taking the lead to be able to sit in the chair, then her, then me. Then I could close the door. It was tight, y'all!

After we chatted briefly, I had her lie on her back on the table. I invited her husband, who was already looking at his watch, to stand and assess her with me—to tell me what he saw.

He described his wife as lying "bent" like a banana, grayish in color, cool to the touch. I explained craniosacral therapy: a hands-on treatment with very light pressure. She was concerned because of the pain of CF/FM. Her husband watched as I worked silently on his wife. I made no sudden movements, just allowing the cerebrospinal fluid from the interior of the brain to flow more freely down the spinal cord to nourish the nerves feeding the organs and muscles.

When I was finished, I asked him to assess her with me again. His eyebrows went up as he exclaimed she was lying straight with better color (no longer gray) and warmer to his touch. I hadn't moved her at all!

I asked her how she felt in that moment.

"Fine," she replied.

Was she in any pain in that moment, I asked?

She started to talk about the future, so I brought her back to that moment. No pain. Muscles, joints, gut? No pain!

I helped her sit up and asked the same questions. She felt fine with **no pain anywhere**. I gave her a simple diet plan, made an appointment for two weeks away, and gave her one piece of homework: she needed to decide if she wanted to LIVE… or not! If she chose to live, she would keep her appointment with me and I would help her reverse her chronic diseases of exclusion (all labs and imaging say she's "fine" when she clearly was not).

If she chose to continue with her current life habits, I added, she should cancel her next appointment and stop calling for help that she didn't actually want.

She canceled two days before her next appointment.

What possible conclusions might we draw, Reader?

Her condition was serving her somehow. Ooh! Maybe it was even keeping her husband with her. Oof.

That's what I figured. He drove her to her appointments. She'd already told me on the phone that he did everything because she could not—shopping, cooking, cleaning. (Maybe he hired help.) What if she believed he'd divorce her if she were "capable" of self-care? Belief drives behavior, Reader! A bit later, we'll look at more reasons why people might choose chronic disease management over vibrant health.

Building A Strong Foundation

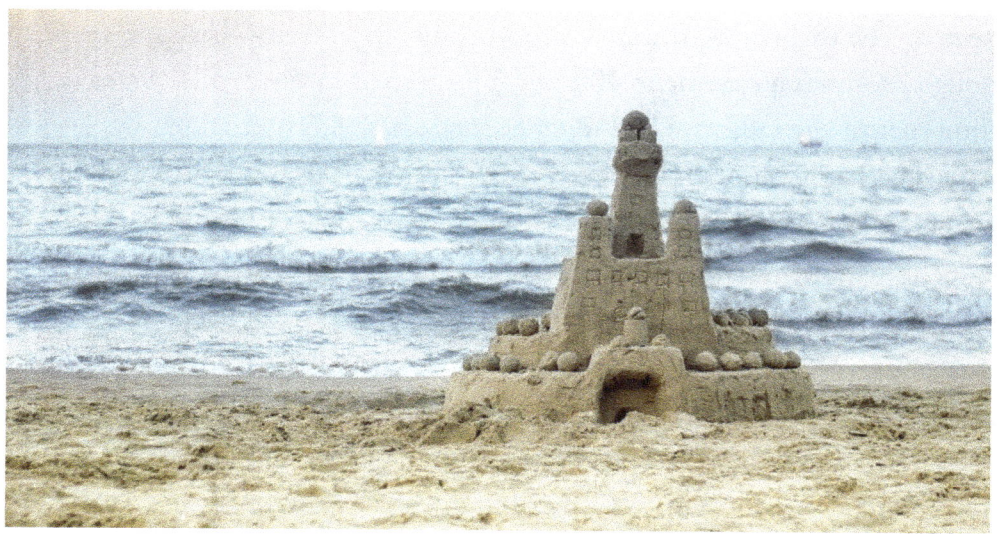

(Picture taken from Microsoft 365)

How fabulous is this sand castle? And what'll happen to it when the tide comes in or the rain falls?

I want better for you. In order for you to have a strong foundation, *you* have to want better for you! *You* will have to "lay the groundwork" (foundation) for better health. I'm just providing the blueprint.

Reader, you are *important*! You are here for a *reason*! I firmly believe that you have a *purpose* on this planet. Let's get you into the best health—physically, emotionally, mentally and spiritually—so you've got the strength, stamina, energy, and passion to become who you were meant to be and do all you were created to do! "We were meant to *live!*" sings my favorite band (Switchfoot).

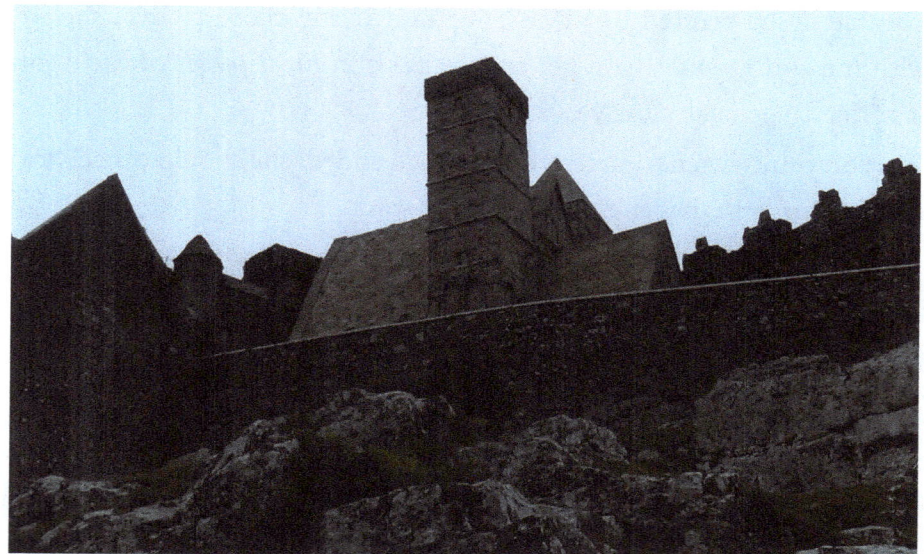

This castle is stone built on rock in Tipperary, Ireland. (Photo by me!)

I have a few exercises to help get us started on solid footing, like that castle above. When the "tide comes in," the rain falls hard, the going gets rough… this castle will remain. It already has through many centuries. Let's ensure your foundation is as secure as can be.

Exercise One

List your Core Four priorities for this season of your life, in order of importance. For example, mine are:

1. God, our relationship (spiritual health)
2. Me (physical, emotional, mental health)
3. My relationships with my immediate family members (husband, sons)
4. My work (writing, teaching, mentoring, caring for others, non-profit work)

This sounds incredibly self-centered, doesn't it? *Aren't we supposed to put everybody else before us?* When I did that, I burned out. I realized I'd put my work or my spouse in spot number one, with fairly disastrous results.

The way I figure it, when God is on His Throne (#1), I'm not trying to sit there, so I'm already in a much more reasonable posture. The closer I am to Him (#2), really, the better my life goes.

As marvelous as my spouse is, he's not ultimately responsible for me. I am solely responsible for my choices: what I eat, drink, think, meditate upon, etc.

The kids are grown, but they're "mine" and I love them forever, making myself available to them when they make a request to spend time with me, no matter the reason.

My work shifts and changes with seasons and perceived needs. This season of my life allows me to teach, write, take care of people, speak, and travel.

These Core Four make up the bulk of my life. Yours doesn't have to look anything like mine; we're different, you and I. We can have different priorities. The point here is for you to get clear on yours!

1. Most important:
   _____

2. Second most important:
   _____

3. Third most important:
   _____

4. Fourth most important:
   _____

The second part of this exercise is to show your Core Four, in order, to your best friend. Ask the person who knows you really well if you are living your life in a way that highlights your priorities in that order. If your very best friend hears you say you think you live one way (by reading your list), but in reality, they see you living out something different, it's time for you to either be truthful about what really is important to you or to change your ways. In other words, *walk your talk*. Be congruent in thought, word, and deed. Dis-ease loves to breed in incongruity!

We talked about costs earlier. Other costs in disease reversal include the time/energy of putting yourself in your Core Four, thinking differently, and finding a community to support and cheer you on. Sometimes the bigger obstacles come from within. You might have a problem with either your own faulty thinking or default ways of living. Sometimes the people we live with can't comprehend why we would want to disrupt their lives by changing *us*. Anyone with me on this one?

Exercise Two

Determine your short-term and your long-term motivations. The best short-term motivator is typically **fear**. Given the disease you're curious about reversing, what scares you the most about continuing to be medically managed, or continuing to choose to do nothing about it? Jot that down right here because this will help you start your journey.

_____
_____
_____
_____

Next, think about life *without* the limitations of the disease. What do you most want? **Desire** is a very strong motivator over the long haul. Knowing what drives you will help you continue the adventure when the going gets tough, as every good adventure is likely to do.

What I most WANT:

_____
_____
_____
_____

Exercise Three

Take a literal picture of yourself. Get as much of you in the frame as possible, as well as a close-up of your beautiful face. (Please don't argue with me. We're all allowed to have our own opinions, remember? I don't have to see your beautiful face to know you're beautiful, regardless of your own opinion concerning your appearance.)

Along with the picture, create a snap-shot of the totality of you on paper, right now. Write down how you see you. Most of us can start easily enough with all the things that are "wrong," like carrying too much weight, wrinkles galore, sagging skin, discoloration….

Okay, go deeper: What's "wrong" in your body? Blood pressure, cholesterol, glucose too high; constipation, diarrhea, heartburn; recurrent infections; chronic pain, waning sex drive…

Good! Keep going deeper: What's "wrong" in your emotions? Are you depressed too often, anxious too often, easily angered, road rage, crying for no apparent reason, crying and knowing exactly why but cannot resolve the issue…

What's "wrong" in your mind? Include nagging or ruminating thoughts, a "To Do" list that's left half undone each day interfering with sleep, conversations that went badly during the day also interfering with sleep, can't seem to focus during the day, "brain fog"…

Finally, what's "wrong" in your spirit? Self-esteem in the toilet, purposeless in this life, unfulfilled in relationships, restless and irritable, addiction issues, PTSD without PTG (post-traumatic stress disorder without post-trauma growth)…

The next part of the exercise asks you to go back over what you've written and honestly list the "right/good" parts of you, too, starting with the **physical**: natural curls in your hair made even more stunning by the glorious silver and platinum streaks that sparkle in the sunlight, gorgeous eyes, easy smile, a body that's still strong despite years of use...

_____
_____
_____
_____

What's right in your **emotional** range that allows for cleansing tears (because you've got such a big, fluffy, compassionate heart), belly-felt laughter and everything in-between; experiences that, combined with the rest of you, could totally be transformed to help others in similar circumstances...

_____
_____
_____
_____

What are the best things about your **mind?** Is it sharp, well-educated from books and schooling or "street smarts" or both or something else altogether, specific skills and gifts that are useful in service to others, able to "see" what others cannot, or explain difficult concepts in easy-to-understand ways?

_____
_____
_____
_____

Do you have a **spirit** that sings, meets others right where they are in love rather than judgment, speaks up and out for the weak and marginalized, and appreciates beauty and justice?

_____
_____
_____
_____

Are you starting to see how very complex and magnificent you are? How deep and rich your various layers are? You are so much more than the sum of your parts!

We looked at four layers above. Three of those levels cannot be measured, photographed, or "seen." Think about that. Our thoughts are immaterial. So are our emotions. So is the soul and/or spirit. (We'll cover the relevant definitions to make sure we're all on the same page, or at least you'll know what I mean by these words, momentarily.)

Simple math says that three-fourths of who we are is *immaterial*. But humans aren't "simple." We're quite complex.

> Here's a fascinating 1970's short film showing the "power of ten", from our earthly perspective way beyond our own galaxy, then micro-coping down to the hum of a single proton: https://www.youtube.com/watch?v=0fKBhvDjuy0

Astrophysicists say that if we're a microcosm of the universe (or macrocosm), 95 percent of who we are is non-physical (immaterial). Applying that to medicine, we've been trying to manipulate a mere five percent of the human being through chemical agents or surgical procedures, when our suffering often starts in a non-physical location housed within our physical frames.

Have you ever felt your digestion (esophagus, stomach, small intestines) simply STOP, perhaps during a conversation at the table that suddenly "hit a nerve?" That's a complex interplay between your beliefs and another's spoken thoughts, which then spark an emotional response, changing your biochemistry and affecting your nervous system, pushing you out of parasympathetic dominance (rest, digest) and into sympathetic nervous system dominance (fight, flight). In less than a fraction of one second, all this can transpire, absolutely shutting off your digestive capacity.

Was that a physical punch to the gut? No, not at all—but it had the same effect. Likewise, much of our suffering begins on a plane that's not physical. It's as if we're designed as spirit first, wrapped in material body (C.S. Lewis).

Embryologically, we develop from the inner portion of the brain (inside, top) downward and outward. That's how we heal, too. Constantine Hering, MD, the father of American homeopathy, told us his "laws": that we heal from the top down, from the more interior portions to the more external, and in reverse order of how we got sick. See? Here is another place where a Trauma Timeline will come in handy! We can travel backwards in time. While you can't change the circumstances of what happened, you can change your future—to a degree. ☺

Back to the body-wrapped spirit... I believe our physical bodies are our longest-time, closest friends and that they speak to us in the kindest way possible to get our attention, redirecting us to the path of our spirits. At times, my own body has broken. Once, while painting inside a dormer, I bent down to get more paint on the roller, stood up, started walking, and BAM! I slammed my head into the dormer frame and hit the floor. As I was lying on the ground, I heard myself say aloud, "Seriously? You've got to whack me upside the head to get my attention?" Clearly, the answer was "Yes." Unfortunately. Or fortunately—I didn't give myself anything worse than a slight concussion, and I learned new ways of treating brain injury in the process of my own recovery. Bonus!

Here's a pictural description of what I'm trying to describe:

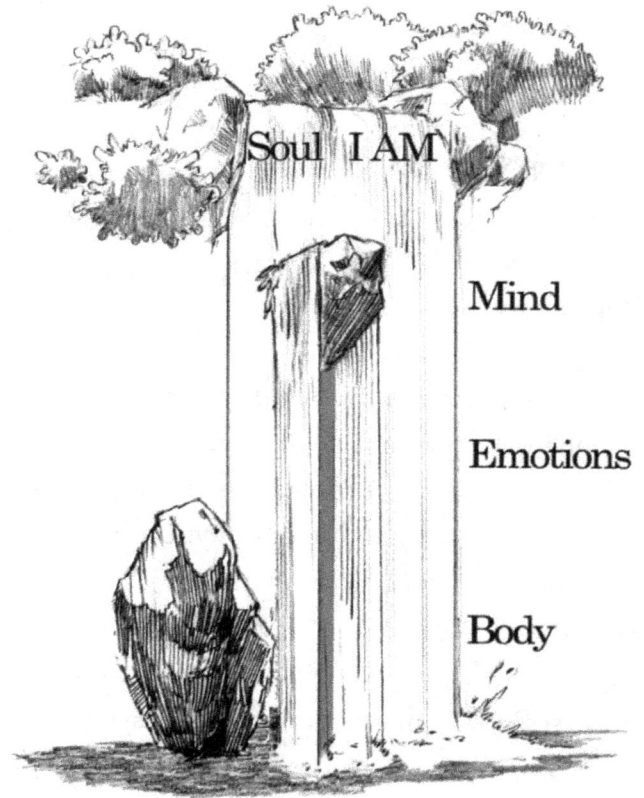

Picture 2 – The Direction of Influence of the four Dimensions of the Whole Person
from Holistic Counseling book - Dr. Moshe
20

This comes straight out of my friend and colleague's book, Holistic Counseling by Moshe Block.

Because we're a little bit different in how we see the world and our places in it, I've altered his illustration a little bit in the next picture.

The way I define things is as follows: Spirit is ever-present, ever flowing, clean and clear! When capitalized, I think of God's Spirit; lower case is my own/your own spirit.

Our souls/spirits interface with Spirit. Ego gets in the way of Spirit's flow. Our thoughts (Mind) can become like the downed trees and rocks impeding Spirit. Our feelings (Emotions) are like the chaotic swirl of water at the base of the waterfall. Our Bodies hold all of this, depicted by the earth. In my schema, Soul represents the combination of Mind + Emotions. Current culture just doesn't talk often about "soul."

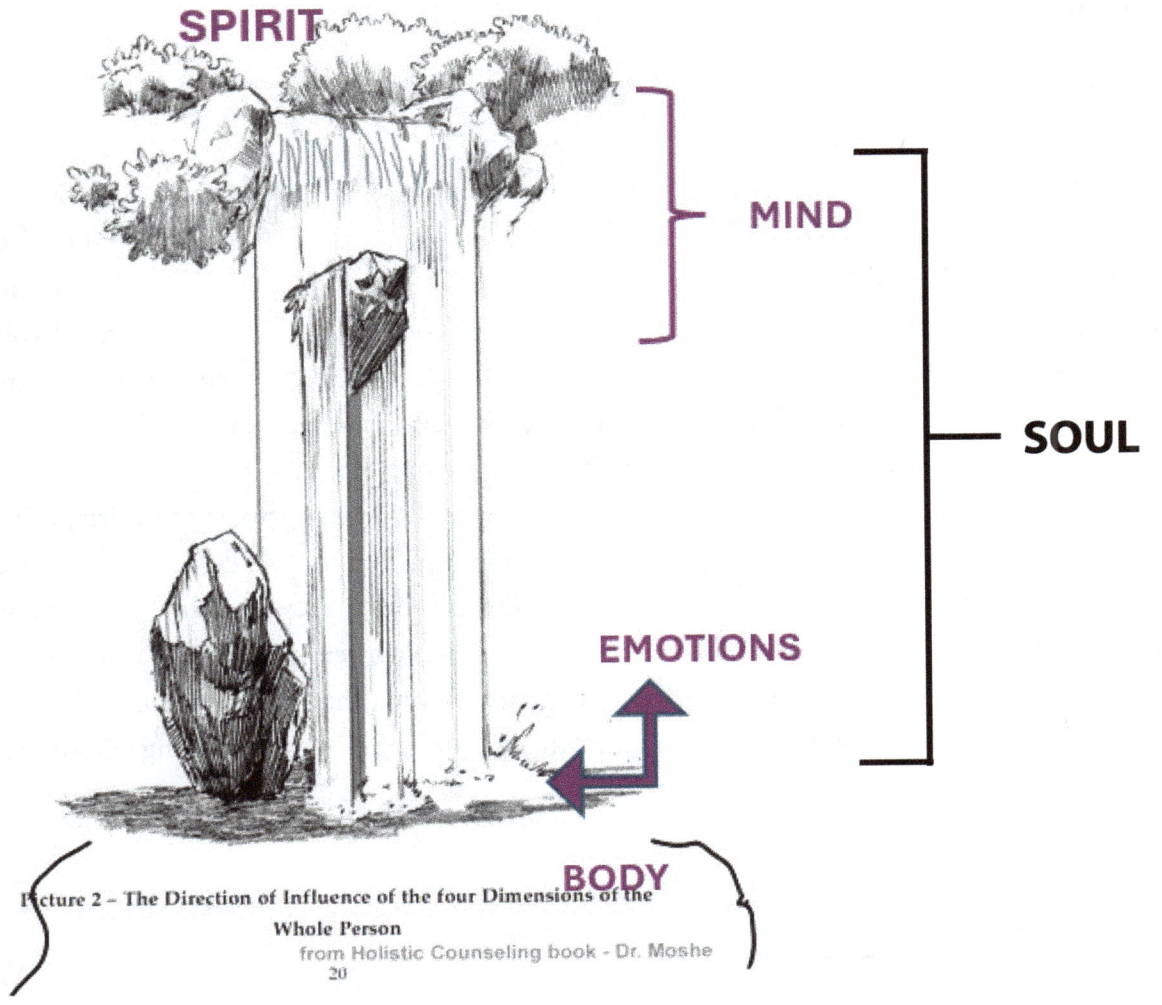

Picture 2 – The Direction of Influence of the four Dimensions of the Whole Person
from Holistic Counseling book - Dr. Moshe

More definitions:

Body: Anatomy, physiology, biochemistry, nutritional status, genetics, epigenetics—Our lifestyle

Emotions: Bliss, ecstasy, the abyss of despair, everything in between, the "ladder" or "atlas" of emotions, stable or not—Our experiences

Mind: What you think, why you think that, our own wills, opinions, biases—Our stories: what we tell ourselves

Spirit: What you believe, why you believe that, purpose/destiny/plan, God in you—Animating force of life

The more we learn, the more we realize how little we actually know. And that's on the *physical plane*—the one we can see and measure, put things into, take things out of! Anyway, I'm open to suggestions. This version helps me help other people, so I'm sticking with it for now.

Don't put off for tomorrow something that you could do *right now*! If you want to reverse chronic disease, it starts with an honest assessment of who you are, where you've been, where you are now, and where you want to go. Which leads us to…

Creating Your Map And Next Logical Steps

Exercise Four

Yet another two-part exercise!

First, write out your "Trauma Timeline" starting with your birth story. What was your mother experiencing while pregnant with you? Where was your birth in relation to other children your mother had? Are you part of a blended family? From your birth story to about age ten, jot down all the things that took you off your perceived trajectory. If you and your best friend at age eight planned your entire lives together, then that friend suddenly and unexpectedly moved away, your eight-year old self was abruptly cut adrift from all those plans. That goes on your "Trauma Timeline." Remember, I love alliteration! Call it simply "Timeline" if you prefer. Just do it, please?

Likewise, jot down all that comes to mind between ages ten to twenty, twenty to thirty, thirty to forty, and all the way up to present. I expect emotions might surface for you during this exercise. When that happens, simply jot down what's coming up. Take a break. Treat yourself with kindness. Come back! Keep going. There's insight for you right around the corner; with insight often comes healing. There's always a nugget of Truth or Treasure in that Trauma that you'll want to hold onto while the drama in the trauma drops away. Sometimes it takes a few episodes of revisiting said trauma to debride and actually heal an ugly wound.

Birth story:

_____
_____
_____
_____

Childhood:

_____
_____
_____
_____

Tweens and Teen years:

_____
_____
_____
_____

Disease Reversal: Hypertension, Dyslipidemia, Type 2 Diabetes

Twenties:
_____
_____
_____

Thirties:
_____
_____
_____

Forties:
_____
_____
_____

Fifties:
_____
_____
_____

Sixties:
_____
_____
_____

Seventies:
_____
_____
_____

Eighties:

___

Nineties:

___

Part two. When you've finished with the "Trauma Timeline" all the way up to the present-day you, pull out your medical files and list in a different pen color when you were given medical diagnoses, i.e., high blood pressure, diabetes, tonsillitis. Add interventions, i.e., prescriptions, procedures. Be as specific as possible, listing the prescription name, dose, and duration, along with the dates used. If changes to the drug occurred over time, or you switched from one drug to another in a similar class, write that down. All this detail will inform your practitioner how to better care for you. It also shows your direction of healing, preparing you for what's coming back around again for resolution.

Here's extra space for your Medication History:

___

TANGENT: Top Ten Myths and Stumbling Blocks

Let's see if any of these myths resonate with you. You might need to remove these obstacles in your path to vibrant wellness:

1. "It's in my genes!"
    a. Reader, dearest, you have control over 70 to 90 percent of how your genes express themselves by how you choose to live! Genes cannot code for disease; they can, in the absence of necessary nutrients, code as best they can under the circumstances, which may produce something less than vibrant health. Whether disease gets turned "on" or "off" depends, to a very large extent, on *you*.

Disease Reversal: Hypertension, Dyslipidemia, Type 2 Diabetes

   b. What did you get from your parents other than their genetic contributions? You got their coping strategies, their biases, their belief system, their relationship with money, their eating habits…. In short, you got their *lifestyle*! And you thought it was "normal." (SPOILER ALERT: "Normal" does not mean "healthy!" Maybe you were raised in a "normal" home; I'm teaching you how to break out of that mold and be "healthy!")
   c. When we choose to change our lifestyles—moving away from a style of inflammation and depression and stress and dis-ease, toward mobility and clear thinking and health promotion—the disease-state simply has nothing left to feed on, literally and figuratively!
2. "Healthy foods don't taste good."
   a. Taste buds can be reminded to love healthy food. You are designed to eat food that is real, not processed, stripped of nutrients, and pumped full of chemicals intended to "hook" you.
   b. Let's call an addiction what it is—an addiction! You may well be addicted to chemicals, fats, sugars, salt. Getting you hooked is part of the food industry's *job* these days!
   c. Once you clean up your diet and offer your amazing body the proper fuel it needs to work efficiently, it will!
3. "All my favorite foods would have to go away in order for me to get healthy."
   a. Aha! You at least understand that your foods are causing you to be unhealthy. Excellent—you're off to a great start!
   b. There's always a less-toxic alternative to be found. Take the wrapper of whatever you think you can't live without to the local health food store and ask one of their employees to help you find a substitute.
   c. Over time, you'll change your mind, along with your tastebuds, and opt for even healthier foods.
4. "It's too hard."
   a. Ever heard the quote, "Nothing in the world is worth having or worth doing unless it means effort, pain, difficulty…."? (Theodore Roosevelt) Your *one life* is *precious*. Your *one body* is *priceless*. **You are worth this effort!**
   b. I have helped countless others **reverse their diseases**; I can help you, too.
   c. I've reversed my own disease by changing my own life. I used to eat fast food most days, drink soda all day long, and eat candy bars nearly every afternoon. If I can change—and write the curriculum to teach doctors how to counsel other people to change—*you* can change, too!
5. "Eating healthy is too expensive."
   a. In the beginning, as you're reading labels and learning to shop differently, yes, it will be more expensive. It will cost money, time, and energy. That will shift as you're able to recognize a "safe" food item in the warehouse setting or mega-store.

b. How expensive is your disease? **Type 2 diabetes**, in this country, runs about $250 per month in out-of-pocket expenses. Not to mention the emotional, mental, and physical strain, potential loss of work due to complications or even routine monitoring of diabetes (despite the medications). And that's not including being passed over for a promotion because you've missed too many days from work or your performance has suffered due to the strain of having diabetes. And we're not counting missing events with family and friends—and dying earlier than expected.

c. If you're self-employed, the burden of having any chronic disease and its projected progression can be even *more* expensive.

6. "I'm too far gone/I have too many diseases to reverse anything."
    a. I'd be ever-so-curious to have a conversation with you, to hear your story and understand why you think this (and the next myth on this list). I have seen what conventional medicine deems "medical miracles" and I've witnessed them *on a daily basis* with my desperately ill patients/clients. Type 2 diabetes is a piece of cake (pun intended) compared to other diseases I've helped people **reverse**. If you happen to have the exceptionally *common* cardiometabolic triad: **high blood pressure, high cholesterol,** and **type 2 diabetes**? No problem*!*
    b. Got depression and/or anxiety and/or sleep issues and/or erectile dysfunction to accompany the diabetes? No problem*!* Really, these separate diagnoses are all related*!*
    c. You *may be* "too far gone." But since I'm the subject matter expert in this, how about I weigh in on the truth of the matter before you give up?

7. "Even though your plan sounds good and the evidence seems solid, reversing disease may work for others, but it likely won't work for me."
    a. See above (Myth #6).
    b. No, seriously!
    c. What do you have to lose, at this point? *Right:* Your eyesight, your sex life, your kidneys, your *limbs*! I am throwing you a virtual *lifeline*! Please think enough of yourself to grab hold. (Reader, some people's identity is so wrapped up in a given diagnosis that to heal them would destroy their toxic current way of living.)

8. "I don't know enough about this!"
    a. You didn't *know* that most diseases were lifestyle driven and that changing the lifestyle alters the disease process and outcome. Now you do!
    b. Ignorance may be "bliss," but it can still *kill* you! (Eighteenth-century English poet Thomas Gray wrote: "Where ignorance is bliss, 'tis folly to be wise.'")
    c. "Knowledge is *power!*" (Sir Francis Bacon, circa 1597)—but only if you *apply* your new knowledge to your life! Keep reading; keep learning. When we stop growing, we start dying.

9. "I should eat this food and take this medicine—because the media told me to!"
   a. Our culture promotes poor health with direct-to-consumer pharmaceutical advertising—ads with strong emotional hooks that encourage drug-seeking behavior (*"Ask your doctor if this drug is right for you"*).
   b. Our culture also promotes chemical-filled "foods," "fast" foods, "junk" foods, overly processed foods, and "food stuffs." (*What even IS that?* Whatever it is, it isn't *food!* Don't eat it!)
   c. Vote with your shopping dollars! Push back against this growing "sick-care" model by refusing to listen to the media! Let's *change the culture* to one that values *health*!

Our final myth is this:

10. "This can't be true if conventional medicine doctors don't know about it!"
    a. You were probably told you'd have this disease for the rest of your life, that there is no "cure." For *them*, your disease *is* "incurable." But I'm *not* one of them! I understand the drugs even *better* than they do. I also know a different way to view the body and engage it to heal itself. We are, after all, created/designed for *health*!
    b. You are probably aware that the medical system is broken, and that doctors are trained to *manage* disease, not *reverse* it.
    c. You were probably *not* told to change your lifestyle for a different outcome, or that the drugs used to treat ("manage") high blood pressure, cholesterol abnormalities, and/or type 2 diabetes are supposed to be used *in conjunction lifestyle changes, or after lifestyle efforts have failed.*

That was a bit of a rant. Hopefully, it helped more than a few of you.

Naturopathic Medicine's History And Philosophy, and Why This Stuff Matters

More than a 130 years ago, my profession "became." An immigrant from Europe, Benedict Lust, ventured into New York City, got trampled by a horse, and went back home to Germany to recover. He was healed by a priest, Father Kneipp, through proper nutrition (*even back then!*), water therapies, simple herbal remedies and prayer, all in a natural setting of sunlight and open air. Young Benedict, once healed, studied water therapies under Father Kneipp, who then sent him back to the growing country of the United States of America to spread the good news of clean, healthy living, which is a birthright of all humanity, and especially to those of us who believe we're made in God's very image.

Lust studied every medicine imaginable, including graduating from both conventional and osteopathic medical schools, and then cobbled together the "best of the best" in his opinion for HEALTH: nutritionists, herbalists, exercise therapists/hygienists, homeopaths, and mind-body practitioners. He combined these modalities or therapies under the new name "Naturopathy."

Lust opened the first medical school of naturopathy and the first sanatorium, an inpatient clinic focused on getting people vibrantly WELL, in New York. The next naturopathic school would open in Chicago under the leadership of medical doctor Henry Lindlahr. He'd been a skeptic, but naturopathy healed him of the then-terminal diagnosis of type 2 diabetes. Lindlahr would codify naturopathic practice.

According to Dr. Lindlahr, there are three primary reasons why disease takes place:
1. Lowered vitality. (Encompasses body, emotions, mind, spirit)
2. Abnormal composition of blood and lymph.
3. Accumulation of waste matter, morbid materials, and poisons.

But why? How? Any of the three factors listed above tend to lower, hinder, or inhibit normal function (harmonious vibration) and engender and promote the destruction of living tissues. –Taken from Lindlahr's book, *Nature Cure*.

In order to correct the three primary reasons for disease, Dr. Lindlahr determined these six pillars of health:
1. Establish normal surroundings and natural habits of life in accord with Nature's Laws.
2. Economize the Vital Force.
3. Build up the blood on a natural basis; that is, supply the blood with its natural constituents in right proportions.
4. Promote elimination of wastes and poisons without in any way injuring the human body.
5. Correct mechanical lesions.
6. Arouse the individual to the highest possible degree to the consciousness of personal accountability and the necessity of intelligent personal effort and self-help.

I love that last one!

About thirty years ago, naturopathic doctors Jared Zeff and Pamela Snider wrote the Therapeutic Order for our present-day profession, which spans from teaching our patients the Determinants of Health all the way up to frank suppression of symptoms, chemo/radiation and palliative care (for patients who are dying). We're trained to use the appropriate tools all along the "steps" of the Therapeutic Order (as I've drawn them here).

You can probably see the similarity between Lindlahr's thinking and the ordered approach Zeff and Snider used. One of the delights of being a naturopath, in my opinion, is that we have the fluidity of utilizing various steps simultaneously for the most efficient positive patient outcome. In my office, for example, my client may have been given the very same homework I'm about to give you and might have already started adding a few healthy habits to the lifestyle (Therapeutic Order Step 1; Lindlahr 1, 3, 4). While the client is with me, they receive some body work (Therapeutic Order Steps 2, 3, 4; Lindlahr 5) or perhaps some counseling (Therapeutic Order Step 2; Lindlahr 2, 6). I might make an herbal blend or recommend specific teas for my client (Therapeutic Order Steps 1, 3, 4; Lindlahr 3, 4).

Disease Reversal: Hypertension, Dyslipidemia, Type 2 Diabetes

The way I see it, my job is to work myself right out of a job, one patient/client/family at a time!

The Therapeutic Order

- 7 — Suppression, chemo, surgery, palliation
- 6 — Address pathology with pharmaceuticals
- 5 — Address pathology with nutraceuticals
- 4 — Correct structural integrity
- 3 — Address weak/damaged systems
- 2 — Stimulate the inherent self-healing of the body (*Vis*)
- 1 — Remove obstacles to cure; restore/establish determinants of health

Stop the "bad", put in the "good", get out of the way!
- Raise vitality
- Nourish the blood
- Remove the waste

Historically, steps 6 and 7 have been the purview of medical doctors, while steps 3 and 4 are the realm of the new functional/integrative doctors (terms used by medical doctors who stepped outside their educational scope to learn naturopathic tools without the philosophy; now steadily being used by naturopathic doctors). Step 5 is the "meeting ground," so to speak, between the two camps.

Who gets steps 1 and 2? Those steps are **foundational** to health! Without those two often-overlooked steps being addressed, none of the rest of the steps will "hold." Like a house, if you build a groovy spiral staircase, bay windows, and a turreted balcony on the fourth floor before digging a stable foundation, the whole structure will collapse.

I happen to live in the coolest house ever. I have spiral stairs from the basement to the top (fourth) floor, sliding panels, rooms off other rooms, a massive front porch, a top floor balcony, and a back porch.

Over the past forty years of the structure's existence, the spiral stairs have become scoliotic. Chiropractor friends and bodyworkers have much to say upon entering my eclectic home. When I teach the Therapeutic Order, I now include a picture of my unique staircase to accentuate the point that, if the patient walks in with a high level of pathology, something that warrants high-level intervention, by all means, take those stairs two at a time! Once stabilized, however, ensure that every one of those stairs is touched firmly—with corrective action, if necessary.

At my house, we run up crooked stairs *all day long*. But it's dangerous to consider skipping steps on the way down. The distance between some of the steps is inconsistent with adjacent steps; the pitch is different between steps, and some have repositioned themselves underneath an adjacent step. (We are working with a brave contractor who's devising our "next steps." Hah! See what I did there?)

Supplements

The short piece on nutraceuticals is that many of our beloved providers have been purchased by corporations to whom I wouldn't choose to give my money; quality is slipping, as is therapeutic benefit. And, when we manipulate one element in the body, we shift something else downstream. (Like MTHFR "mutations" being supplemented with methylated folic acid, then adversely impacting the COMP pathway. Not to mention that folic acid is a cheap imitation of the methyl-rich folate we find in natural foods and has growing evidence of being a poison to the human body. See? In order to educate about the supplement industry's ingredient list, a whole 'nother book is indicated!)

It's the same in medicine. If I skip teaching you how to live healthily/healthfully—if you never learn the **determinants of health**—at best, you're relegated to a lifetime of pills, in the form of pharmaceuticals or nutraceuticals. Nutraceuticals come with their own risks. Everybody seems to be looking for the "magic bullet," be it in the latest and greatest prescription drug on the market, an herbal blend, odd cosmetic, gadget, or "reason why." We want *one thing* to "fix" *all the things* that cause us suffering.

SPOILER ALERT: There is no "magic bullet" anywhere.

But… There *are* "miraculous bebes!" (Maybe you know these as "BBs"—little metal balls shot from small guns. Remember the kid in "A Christmas Story" who desperately wanted a bebe/BB gun? His parents kept telling him "no" because he'd shoot his eye out?) As you read the following, feel free to put a check mark by the behaviors you've already claimed for your own personal habit (high five!), circle another 2-3 that make good sense to you to start doing now, and leave the rest for your next steps. As you apply each good habit, you'll notice a modicum of improvement in your health. You'll "feel" better, generally. Sleep will become more restful. Your mind will calm. Your emotions will be less volatile. Over time, you'll be able to look back and see a large measure of improvement from the combination of "all the things."

We are simply gorgeous in our very complex design! Don't be fooled by advertisements of a quick fix by the "one thing."

One *more* thing: Now's a good time to revisit the snapshot you took of yourself at the beginning of this book. There are pages at the end for you to either copy or use to log your daily blood pressure (Appendix A), daily blood glucose (Appendix C), or quarterly cholesterol readings (get your own copies to keep from your doctor). These objective measurements will be pivotal in your future conversation with your prescriber.

Once you start implementing the listed "miraculous bebes," you must be keeping track of both your *objective signs* and *subjective symptoms* of disease to know when you're becoming over-medicated and need to speak with your prescriber!

Objective signs: Things you can measure.

- To monitor **high blood pressure**, take **daily blood pressure readings**. Sit comfortably with your feet flat on the floor for about five minutes at about the same time every day. Take your blood pressure once. Record it. If you want to get fancy, take a once daily "rolling" blood pressure. (Appendix A)
- For **cholesterol abnormalities**, get a routine lipid panel. Please make that a **quarterly lipid panel** once you start making healthier choices by requesting that your provider authorize a lipid panel every three months.
- For **type 2 diabetes**, use your **daily blood sugar readings** (Appendix C) **or continuous glucose monitoring** (CGM) device. Ensure your CGM is in correct position to provide useful data.

Subjective symptoms: Things you feel/sense internally.

- For **hypertension**, when you start becoming over-medicated, you may experience episodes of low blood pressure when you move quickly from a seated position to standing, or from lying down to sitting up quickly. It could feel like dizziness or lightheadedness. Take your blood pressure when these sensations occur!
- For **dyslipidemia**, when you start becoming over-medicated, you may have more muscle aches/pains, an increase in loose stools, cramping, fatigue, decreased sex-drive, and/or foggy thinking. If you have three consecutive days of any combination of these symptoms, please call your doctor for an appointment plus a fasting blood draw to determine your lipid status.
- For **type 2 diabetes**, your close friends/family will likely be the first to recognize when you start becoming over-medicated. Your moods will probably shift a bit more quickly and with greater intensity. Any deviation away from normal blood sugar levels can push a person into depression and/or anxiety. You may also feel weak, wiped out, even "hangry" (hungry and angry, suddenly and rather strongly). When this happens, check your blood glucose RIGHT THEN! And get a healthy snack.

You need to know and do these things NOW. I'll remind you again as we go along. My job is to educate you. Your job is to make the positive changes to your life that will then start the disease reversal process.

We're together in this book, but you're not my client. I'm not monitoring your progress. I've stated it already, but I'll state it again:

**DO NOT TAKE YOURSELF OFF
YOUR PRESCRIPTION MEDICATION!**

Collaborate with your prescriber. Tell your doctor what changes you're making and how your objective and subjective signs and symptoms are also changing.

If your prescriber is unwilling to work with you for freedom from disease and the broken system, find another practitioner. Would you keep a plumber who insisted you keep the leaky faucet so he'd stay in your service? Doctors may go to school longer, but they're still hired professionals like plumbers and electricians (the medical specialty of cardiology is actually split along those lines, interestingly enough). You get my point.

Are you ready? Let's GO!

Starting With The Physical Body: Food, Water, Movement, Sleep

For many of you, this will be a big reminder of what you already "know" is true and right. While knowledge is power, it's only useful when applied to your life! Please move your "knowing" down from your brain into your cells. *Do these things!*

You're now familiar with the costs associated with medical management. There are costs associated with disease reversal, too. The most challenging may be prioritizing your health—not just until the disease reverses, but to keep it gone, too.

Other costs include: an initial increase in your food bill. When folks fail in a plan for better health, it's due to time, energy, or money, so I want to set your expectations right up front. The way you're living is the cause of your suffering, so you know you need to change. Suffering costs you quite a lot over time. Groceries will initially cost more but will decrease over time.

How is that possible? Great question! When you start consuming real food more often than not, you'll feel more satisfied and will therefore eat less. Addictions to things like fats, salts, sweets, and caffeine will make themselves known, providing the excellent challenge of self-control. These addictions wane with time and the associated costs vanish with them.

Food

To decrease frustration, time, and energy costs, I'm going to suggest you start shopping at one of the following. I'm listing these in my order of "safest preference:"

1. Your backyard garden. No more herbicides, pesticides, or fungicides. Choose heritage seeds and plantings.
2. Local Consumer Supported Agriculture (CSA). Get to know your local regenerative farmers!
3. Local health food store
4. AzureStandard.com is an online option for obtaining regenerative foods delivered by truck nationwide.
5. National health food stores such as Whole Foods Market, Trader Joe's, Sprouts.
6. "Natural" sections inside "regular" grocery stores and mega-stores.

Shopping at these locations makes label-reading much easier, saving time and energy at the trade of increased cost.

If you live in a *food desert*—they exist all over our resource-rich country— with few available food sources, your only option could be the "dollar" store around the corner. You'll have to read more labels and put more things back on the shelf if you try to find healthy food there.

But rest assured, lifestyle changes are still possible! If you have computer access, I'll bet Azure Standard has a truck route through or close to your food desert. You can order regeneratively farmed foods from https://www.azurestandard.com/ (Want a discount? Use my code: "Monarch2024".)

When conventional medicine failed me, I started a self-study on what else was "out there." What did humans do in the past to remain healthy? There was a time when doctors were paid only when they kept their patients well! I discovered real food was a basic tenet of health. (*Shocker!*)

Reading the labels on my "food" choices was a fabulous first step to better health. Sugar water was literally my first food—from the hands of a stranger, no less. I learned that as part of researching my birth story. I very quickly became aware of a deeply ingrained sugar addiction.

In my adult quest for health, first, I switched from cookies loaded with ingredients I couldn't pronounce to cookies with legible and recognizable ingredients. Next on the cookie journey, I only ate half the pack over the course of a twelve-hour shift at the pharmacy, rather than the entire bag. I worked the cookie habit all the way down to two cookies only per shift. At this point in my life, if I want a cookie, I make a general announcement to the family which is usually met with one of the cooks in my household baking cookies.

Someone else is baking you cookies? Yes, Reader! And scones! My life is truly sweet. I do grind the ancient grains for the in-house baker.

The point to the story is, when we cook our own food, it's much cleaner! A typical cookie is not likely to ever be considered "healthy," but a less toxic version of whatever you're consuming now is a wonderful step in the right direction.

As you start to diminish and even break your own food addictions, you'll buy less, reducing your overall grocery bill. You'll dine out far less, choosing independently-owned, quality-focused (and probably *more* expensive) restaurants for special occasions. You will still spend less overall while gaining more enjoyment from the experience.

Seriously, eat *real* food. Read every label on everything you put in your mouth or onto your skin. Your skin happens to be a very large organ of both absorption and elimination. If you cannot, with confidence, pronounce each ingredient in a food or cosmetic product, put it back on the shelf and choose again. Better yet, consume products that don't require an ingredient list. Shop the perimeter of the grocery store, focusing on fresh produce; wild-caught, cold-water fish; and local grass-fed/finished lean meats.

The Environmental Working Group offers lists of organically grown foods shoppers can buy to replace the "Dirty Dozen" (most contaminated) produce, as well as the list of food that isn't typically tampered with, which they call the "Clean Fifteen." They can also point you to the least toxic seafood options—without heavy metals and radioactive metabolites—as well as less toxic skin care products.

Here are some of the worst offenders in our foods:

- **Hydrogenated oils and *trans* fats.** Our bodies *require* fat. Our brains are 55 percent fat! But what we need are *cis*-fats. These are wiggly, jiggly fats with lots of double chemical bonds. They are very easily stackable, like spoons in a drawer, yet highly unstable when exposed to ambient air.

    Take fish, for example. If you've ever gone fishing and caught a fish, you might have noticed that there's nothing "fishy smelling" about that fish; rather, it smells like the water it just left. It's not until the fish has been lying in the bottom of the boat, exposed to the oxygen in our air, that it starts to smell "fishy." The fresh fish is high in lovely *cis*-fats that become rancid very quickly when out of the water and exposed to the air.

    Hydrogenated oils are altered so that chemically, the double bonds are changed to single bonds, with lots of hydrogen molecules attached. (In the flatware analogy, the spoons start to look more like forks on both ends.) Food scientists do this to make foods more shelf-stable.

    A *trans*-fat continues the alteration by twisting the structure from a "C" shape to something more like an "S." (Now the spoon-to-fork is more like a bent double-ended fork with bent tines. Definitely not "spoon-able!") This shape is the most marketable because of its long shelf life—but it's also the least digestible.

    Fresh grains also have a marketability problem: Once they are milled into flour, they become rancid quickly. Freshly milled grains are meant to be purchased and eaten within a matter of days to weeks. No one wants to buy moldy, rancid flour! And no one wants to send moldy flour overseas to our soldiers engaged in war, who have limited access to refrigeration of foods.

    During the second World War, millers started separating out the bran and germ from the rest of the flour. The remaining flour was quite stable in transit and could sit on a market shelf for months without going rancid or getting moldy. *Awesome, right?* No. Awful.

    More than 90 percent of the *nutrition* in grains comes from the bran and the germ! But, hey! Our US government, after stripping out more than thirty nutrients from our flours—which are used to make breads, pastas, cookies, cakes, crackers, etc.), decided food manufacturers should put back four to six synthetic chemical substitutes: **vitamin B1 (thiamin), B2 (riboflavin), B3 (niacin), and (in the 1970s) folic acid**. Some manufacturers also add **iron and calcium**. Our government calls these flours "enriched." (*Wait. They stripped out thirty-some natural nutrients, added back only four to six—and those were made in a laboratory—and that's "enriched?"* Yes, my dear Reader. But it gets worse.)

    Next, people who made and sold flour opted to **bleach** all flour, because "white" flour was more aesthetically pleasing than "tan" flour. Mold doesn't thrive in a bleached environment, either. Bleaching also helps the flour "age" faster, making the baked product light and fluffy. (*Wait! Wouldn't aging the flour diminish what nutrition might still be in it?* Ooh! You are catching on quickly! YES!)

Bottom line: Commercial white flour has had almost all its natural nutrition stripped out. Choose unbleached whole grain flours in all foods. Pay extra for real food. What if you miss breads, pastas, cookies, cakes, and crackers? Make your own "junk" food with health-promoting ingredients. You'll eat less of it and it won't be "junk!"

- **Chemical sugar substitutes**: Saccharin, aspartame, and acesulfame K (Ace-K) are foreign substances to our complex systems. Our phenomenal immune systems go into action when foreign invaders enter us, whether the invader is a bacterium, a viral entity, a fungal spore, or a chemical. Chemical sweeteners have been linked to cancer (saccharin), phenylketonuria (aspartame) and nervous system damage due to frank toxicity (all three).

  Chemical sweeteners are marketed to those already diagnosed with **type 2 diabetes and obesity**, but you'll notice that the biggest people in the room are drinking diet drinks. Getting rid of something that was never meant to be in the system to begin with is rather difficult. When the proverbial closets for storage are full, the body makes more. (*Dare I ask what the body's closets are?* Fat cells! *Dang.*)

  Bottom line: If a sweetener is made in a lab, leave it alone. Choose smaller amounts of natural, close-to-nature sweeteners like local honey, grade B maple syrup, black strap molasses (an acquired taste, for sure, but nutritious), and raw, non-GMO cane sugar.

- **Sodium benzoate**: This very common preservative is a known tumor-potentiator, a substance that can encourage tumor growth. Sodium benzoate is in nearly every acidic dark beverage on the shelf, including juices, sodas, and liquid supplements. The risk of tumor formation/growth is actually higher when vitamin C is present in the same food! Avoid sodium benzoate if you're cutting back on growing tumors, both benign and malignant.

- **Sodium nitrite/nitrate**: This is a preservative used in making lunch meats. It causes preferential damage to the heart muscle. Those of you with **high blood pressure**, beware of your sodium nitrite/nitrate intake!

- **High-fructose corn syrup** (HFCS): Corn syrup is made from corn starch and is quite sweet. High-fructose corn syrup is made using genetically modified enzymes to convert much of the inherent glucose molecules in the genetically modified corn to fructose molecules. Seventy pounds of corn can be converted to about thirty-two pounds of HFCS—enough to sweeten 372, twelve-ounce cans of soda (thirty-nine grams each)! While every cell in our bodies can utilize and metabolize sucrose, the liver is the only organ that can metabolize fructose. If you're dealing with **high cholesterol**, you especially need to avoid HFCS! https://www.fooducate.com/community/post/The-Secrets-of-Manufacturing-High-Fructose-Corn-Syrup/57A3487D-2F7C-225A-49CF-A4C49EB02574

- **Artificial colors/flavors**: If it's artificial, it's not recognized in the body. If it's not recognized in the body, it becomes waste material. To many, that waste material is *toxic*. Many artificial colors and flavors are petrochemical byproducts, often adhered to aluminum. Consider ending the assault to your immune system and your brilliant brain by refusing to ingest any more artificial anythings.

Once you're in the habit of avoiding the above worst offenders, you'll have dropped away the lesser offenders.

Bottom line: If you can't pronounce a food ingredient or don't know what it is, it's not food. Another way to look at this is to ask yourself: "Would my grandparents have recognized this as food?"

If you avoid all the toxins listed above, what's left to eat? Here are some tips about new, healthy habits in your choice of produce and meat:

- Aim for five different vegetables and two fruits daily. Choose mixed colors: red, orange, yellow, green, blue, purple, and black. You'll note that all the colors of the rainbow are listed except indigo. That's because I can recognize blue foods; I can recognize purple. But what in nature is indigo and edible? Black is the "wild card"—things that appear black on the outside but smash into some other color on the inside, like black olives, black berries, black currants, black grapes. Eat these when you're running low on one of the other colors. Feel free to eat *more* than five servings of veggies daily but keep the fruits to a maximum of two servings. Fructose (fruit sugar) can only be metabolized by the liver, remember?

- If you eat beef, make it grass-pastured beef only. (*How do I know if I'm cleared for beef?* I'll delve more deeply into this under "*Advanced Topics.*" For now, focus on *clean* foods.) Cows are designed to eat grass. When they are allowed to eat according to their design, their meat actually gives us a stellar set of the omega-3 fatty acids eicosapentaenoic acid and docosahexaenoic acid (referred to as EPA and DHA for obvious reasons). Beef from such cows is similarly nutritious to wild-caught salmon.

    But when cows are provided with grain rather than grass to eat, their meat contains a high amount of the omega-6 fatty acid arachidonic acid. Humans need and make arachidonic acid. It's super important in our own inflammatory cascade. But when we take in extra arachidonic acid from the outside, our inflammatory cascade gets provoked into action by the food, causing us unnecessary pain!

    For my reading PETA friends (People for the Ethical Treatment of Animals) and vegetarian-for-ethical-reasons readers, you are likely already aware of how our cows and chickens are raised in this country. While I need you to understand that vegetarianism isn't the healthiest way for all people to eat—and too many "vegetarians" also have non-nutritious diets—you may skip the next two paragraphs.

    Cows and chickens are usually raised in "concentrated animal feeding operations—CAFOs. CAFOs are a thing to behold, and I don't mean that in a good way—at all. One viewing was more than enough for me. Multiple critters are caged in a tight space with a feed trough running through the middle. The feed is typically GMO corn laced with antibiotics, steroids, and hormones. The animals are literally crowded together: chickens may be stacked cage upon cage in large, ventilated buildings where they never see the sun or touch or eat grass. Because this causes them stress, they have their beaks and claws clipped off so they can't hurt other chickens in the same or adjacent cages. Cows in CAFOs are seen standing in their own cow-patty muck, flicking feces over themselves and their tight neighbors.

The reason their food is laced with antibiotics is that whenever too many critters are packed into a small space with poor sanitation, disease becomes rampant. Eating animals raised on an antibiotic-laced diet is a bigger factor in antibiotic resistance than taking antibiotics when we are sick (!) because the antibiotics in animal flesh also affect our bodies.

Hormones and steroids are given to cause the animals to grow bigger, faster. Steroids also make it harder to tell if an animal is sick until they're seriously ill. *E. coli*, hepatitis E (new to me, too!), avian flu, MRSA and other highly virulent pathogens are associated with CAFOs. If cows were allowed just *ten days* on grass prior to slaughter—a process called "grass finishing"—that would eliminate about 80 percent of the *E.coli* they harbor! https://pmc.ncbi.nlm.nih.gov/articles/PMC8784678/

Also consider the stress hormones the animals produce by being trapped in such a circumstance. All that anxiety and fear!

Exactly, Reader. That's why we're having this conversation.

Who "owns" our food chain?

As of 2025, the global food system is dominated by three main groups:

- The Seeds & Chemicals owners ("owning" the start of the food chain through patents and tech, even before a seed is planted): Bayer (Monsanto), Corteva, Syngenta, BASF.

- The Traders/Gatekeepers (controlling 70-90% of the global grain trade): Archer Daniels Midland (ADM), Bunge, Cargill, Dreyfus, COFCO.

- The "Big 10" Consumer Giants (processing, distribution): Nestlé, PepsiCo, Unilever, Coca-Cola, Mars, Mondelēz, Danone, General Mills, Associated British Foods, Kellanova (formerly Kellogg's).

Did you know that major corporations now own roughly 80 percent of our food supply? This is another reason to grow your own food, even if you live in a single room with only one window. If you live in a basement apartment, ask if you can grow vegetables in a container on the property. You may have to use fencing to safeguard it from animals.

- **Avoid microwave use.**

ACK! Really? Why?

Reader, what are microwaves?

My favorite browser intelligence says microwaves are a form of electromagnetic radiation.

Good! Where do we use radiation, my friend, and why?

It's used in high-speed data transmission, radar beams, weather forecasting, heating and cooking food...

Good! How about in medicine? Where and why do we use radiation? A different form, but with similar consequences.

Um, cancer care?

Yes! Why?

Because radiation kills cancer?

Yes! How?

Um, I don't know! Just tell me, 'cause you're kinda freaking me out here!

Reader, radiation destroys living tissue once it heats that tissue to 109°F or at a focused intensity. It heats our food (and destroys living tissue) by lodging in fats, sugars, and water and subsequently vibrating those molecules, creating heat.

For the first time ever in human existence, there is a way to heat food from the inside to the outside—which explains why the food doesn't heat evenly. Those vibrating molecules are actually pulled apart, creating heat and deranging the structure of the microwaved food—or the cancerous tumor. Or the developing baby in the womb, or the tiny vessels in the retina of the eye, or the sensitive tissues inside our skulls called the brain!

The atom bomb pulled apart the atom. Microwave ovens pull apart molecules. Cooking from the outside to the inside *denatures* proteins. Cooking from the inside to the outside *deranges* molecular structure. The molecules don't magically pop back into their normal configuration when ("DING") the microwave oven turns off.

You are learning how to buy better quality food to fuel your amazing "machine." By the way, our bodies are a better design than the absolutely best manmade machine on Earth! Please take the extra minutes to denature the proteins in your food by heating from the outside in, rather than deranging the molecules from the inside out. Convection ovens are as compact as microwaves and sit on the counter, unlike the microwave oven placed right at your eye/brain level.

When my parents gifted me a microwave oven upon graduation from pharmacy school, there was a prominent sticker on the front that meant "no pregnant women."

Where has that information gone? I'll bet you can still find it buried deep within the unread pages of your microwave owner's manual. Please, avoid the microwave oven. Keep your brain matter and eyes in good health. Take charge of the things that are within your control. We are all exposed to electromagnetic activity bouncing all around us that we can't control, potentially disrupting our own delicate electromagnetic balance.

Everything is connected to everything else. What impacts one area of your life will, to a degree, impact other parts of your life. Start making positive changes wherever you'd like. Your behavior will change fastest if you can get clear about your beliefs first.

Most of us start at the physical level and ignore the rest until we can't any longer. No matter which aspect of yourself you choose to focus on—physical, emotional, mental, spiritual—you'll start to see improvement in *all* the aspects because *all* those levels are connected and are *you/yours!* Just get started! ☺

For those of you who love lists, the one-page version of this next section may be found at the end of References and Resources.

Checklist for Food Basics

- Eat real food!
- Read labels
    - Avoid *trans*-fats and hydrogenated oils
    - Avoid enriched/bleached grains
    - Avoid chemical sugar substitutes and high-fructose corn syrup
    - Avoid sodium benzoate
    - Avoid nitrites/nitrates
    - Avoid artificial colors/flavors
- Avoid microwaves
- Eat whole grains
- Eat all the colors of the rainbow daily
    - Five or more servings of vegetables
    - No more than two servings of fruits
- Eat grass-pastured beef

Skin Food

Cosmetics are also a big source of toxins. Our skin is a very large organ capable of both absorption and elimination. Here are some of the worst offenders in our skin products:

- **Sodium lauryl/laureth sulfate**: To determine if a product can be labeled "hypo-allergenic," it must pass the "rabbit eye" test. Sodium lauryl sulfate and sodium laureth sulfate both cause irritation to human and rabbit eyes. If a drop of Product A turns the test rabbit's eye red, but a drop of Product B does not redden the other rabbit eye to the same extent, Product B gets the label "hypo-allergenic." (Even with my imagination, I cannot make this stuff up.)

- **Parabens**: These chemicals—including ethyl, methyl, butyl and propyl paraben—all mimic estrogen. (*That's good, right? It keeps the wrinkles at bay?* Initially, yes. But it's not real estrogen; therefore, it becomes, systemically, an *endocrine disruptor*. That's bad, dear Reader.)
- **Petrolatum, mineral oil**: These are two different states of the same petroleum byproduct. Petrolatum is a jelly at room temperature, while mineral oil is a liquid. Because they're waste materials from the petroleum industry, they're exposed to many toxins and require extreme refinement in order to not cause harm to humans.
- **Zinc oxide and titanium dioxide**: I bought into this early on. These are often found in sun-blocking products. Turns out, these minerals get absorbed past the epidermis into the deeper dermal layer, and eventually right into the nucleus of the cell, where they can cause problems within our own DNA. Have you ever noticed that since we started blocking the "harmful" rays of the sun, the incidence of skin cancers has increased?

[This is on that same one-page handout, Naturopathic Basics, at the end of References and Resources.]

Advanced Topics in Food

I promised more information about beef. Grass-pastured beef from a regenerative farmer is key. But only for those who are cleared to eat beef!

Have you ever wondered why the experts can't agree on how best to eat? (I'm getting to the beef, I promise!) Dr. Atkins' plan—low-carb, high protein, carnivore heavy—was opposite of Dr. Ornish's plan (ultra-low fat, vegetarian, no meat), which Dr. Fuhrman ("nutritarian": nutrient-dense vegan, no added salt/oil/sugar) still can't endorse. And these guys are all MDs! What I'm about to lay out for you has been totally thrashed by conventional medical "wisdom," but you're still reading, so here we go.

I teach my clients and patients to eat clean *first*, which fixes all kinds of problems in a fairly short time frame. Then they tend to hit a plateau, which is when I suggest eating according to blood type. Yep! But wait, there's more, because while the blood-type diet is said to work wonders for 85 percent of those who'll give it a try, I happened to fall into the 15 percent who failed at this eating style.

As alluded to before, when I was in my mid-twenties, I had a "Job experience" and became markedly ill. I left the Standard American Diet (*SAD*. Yes, Reader, the Standard American Diet *is* sad. Very SAD!) and then I became vegan for a while and recovered somewhat. (Heck, *anything* is better than the SAD diet!) I tried macrobiotics, but it was too complicated for me then. Raw foodists have the *best* snacks and desserts on the planet, in my opinion, probably because I'm dairy-intolerant and raw eaters are vegans bumped up a notch. No dairy worries at all in that camp!

Improvement came again when I added fish and eggs back into my diet, but I hit another plateau. I didn't fully regain my physical health until I started eating a little bit of red meat each week.

According to the blood-type diet, I should be able to digest dairy from a cow just fine. But I don't! It hurts me three different ways over the course of about a week. Where the blood-type diet shines is that it differentiates between the four different blood types and how foods interact—for good or for ill—with the lectins on the blood cells. (Remember Lindlahr? Reminder below.)

Two generations of brilliant naturopathic physicians have worked on this idea and I've found it to be exceedingly useful in my practice, especially when an old, eclectic naturopathic tool called the "Carroll Method" is overlaid on the blood-type eating plan to remove the "good, healthy" foods that are neither "good" nor "healthy" for a given individual. Once I did this for myself, everything got better—including my mind and my emotional state! Foods and/or food combinations can adversely affect the body, causing rash, gas, bloating, and more. Food can also affect the emotions, contributing to anxiety, depression, irritability, mania, meanness—and the mind, making us forgetful, "foggy," and unfocused.

According to Dr. Lindlahr, there are three primary reasons why disease takes place:
1. Lowered vitality. (Encompasses body, emotions, mind, spirit)
2. **Abnormal composition of blood and lymph.**
3. Accumulation of waste matter, morbid materials, and poisons.

In order to correct the three primary reasons for disease, one of his six pillars of health is **"Build up the blood on a natural basis, that is, supply the blood with its natural constituents in right proportions."**

Healthy blood is tantamount to *health!* I've had some clients/patients receive their medical miracle simply from choosing to eat according to blood type with the Carroll overlay. Others merely improve. ☺

So how does it work? Right, Reader! Thanks for bringing me back to the point.

Drs. James and Peter D'Adamo (father and son, respectively) developed the plans for eating according to blood type. James noted trends in blood type and eating habits around the globe. In his day of practicing naturopathic medicine, nearly everyone knew his/her blood type, as this information was required to obtain a marriage license. That made it easy for him to start noting patterns of optimal health based on blood type. https://www.dadamoinstitute.com/about-blood-type-diet-sub-blood-type-discoveries/

The quick and easy answers to their more complicated descriptions are like this:

Blood type A: At one end of the eating spectrum, people with this blood type thrive on an ovo-pescatarian (eggs and fish) diet. Whole grains, no red meat, occasional poultry. Lots of vegetables. Minimal dairy. Exercise should be low-intensity: walking, stretching, leisurely gardening.

Blood type O: At the opposite end of the eating spectrum are the blood-type O red-meat eaters! *No* grains, lots of vegetables. Dairy will never be a friend. Exercise should be high-intensity, working out until breaking a sweat, daily.

Blood type B: Type B people are in the middle, so balance is key! Some red meat, some whole grains, lots of vegetables. Dairy-friendly. Exercise should be moderate and fun.

Blood type AB: In-between the A and the B: able to have a bite or so of red meat on occasion, but otherwise ovo-lacto-pescatarian (eggs, dairy, and fish), whole grains, poultry. Lots of vegetables. Exercise should be low-to-moderate intensity and enjoyable.

The Rh factor (whether blood type is positive or negative) does not matter for the eating plan.

Now back to beef. You are "cleared" to eat beef if you are blood type O, B, or (in small amounts only) AB. Blood type A folks are *not* cleared to eat beef or lamb or venison or bison or any red meat!

SPOILER ALERT: *Pork* is not listed as a beneficial food for *any* blood type. Any and all parts of the pig fall into the "Avoid" category for every blood type! (Some of you just set this book down. Hmm.)

Those with auto-immune conditions should stay away from beef, because genetic sequencing between cows and humans are too similar, putting a huge burden on the immune system; and those whose Carroll method indicates a *meat intolerance*. (Yes, that can happen.)

Never stop cow dairy cold turkey! Gradually taper off dairy to diminish the chances of a mucous overload. This may seem a random place to leave such advice. I'll disclose the rationale later.

I'm a B blood type. Of all the blood types, I should be best suited for dairy consumption, but that is not the case. Nope. Within twenty minutes of ingesting any cow dairy, my abdomen becomes inflamed, causing me to look suddenly four months pregnant. I experience searing, knife-like pain across the interior of my gut. The next morning, I'm lethargic and depressed and don't want to get out of bed. Toward the end of the week, my skin starts breaking out like I'm fourteen years old again.

My birth story includes being bottle fed and finding out very quickly that I couldn't digest my cow dairy-based formula, which caused disastrous GI upset. So I was switched to soy-based formula—a horrible choice for a B-blood-type baby, but what did my parents know about blood-type eating? Nothing! James D'Adamo was just figuring it out, and Peter was still quite young.

As I grew older, probably about kindergarten age, my parents started feeding me dairy products again. Shortly after that, I started getting sick with throat issues over and over and over again: strep throat, tonsillitis, pharyngitis, laryngitis… with repeated rounds of antibiotics. My tonsils, by the time I had them removed in high school, weren't even formed glandular tissues any longer, they were so diseased. But no one taught me how to live without cow dairy, so my throat issues moved to my sinuses, and repeated rounds of antibiotics were prescribed for my routine bouts of sinusitis. (Sigh. I was a classic textbook case of dairy intolerance as written about in Henry Lindlahr's book!)

In my late twenties, I was traveling on a plane, reading a book on health. This was during my discovery of "Complementary and Alternative Medicine" phase. When we landed, I'd just finished the chapter (in a book I don't remember the title of now) about dairy consumption being the number one suspect in upper respiratory infections. I marked the page for where to start the next chapter and stopped eating dairy for the entirety of my trip… and I was horribly congested the whole time

I was there. I blamed all the snot on the air flight—breathing other people's germs, stuffy airplane interior, dehydration.

Actually, one can only get sick from other people's germs if they happen to be susceptible to those particular pathogens. The strep infections I kept having as a kid were my own throat's strep inhabitants, not other people's streptococcal species. And airplanes have the best and most sophisticated air filters available. I'm pretty sure I was only drinking water at that point in my life, so dehydration probably wasn't the issue.

Horrible Truth

In 2012, neti-pot use came under great scrutiny after two individuals in Louisiana died of a rare brain infection, reportedly caused by using the neti-pot.

A neti-pot is a container that looks a bit like a Hollywood genie bottle. It's used to irrigate the sinuses—great for allergies and sinus infections. The pot itself is not at all dangerous. One cannot jam the spout far enough up one's nostril to pierce the meninges of the brain.

If your local water supply is contaminated, however, putting microbes next to the brain can be lethal. Such was the case in Louisiana. The neti-pot was completely innocent.

This kind of news should never happen in America—that we're dying from contaminated water! Our wastewater collection and recycling centers were never designed for removing the amount of chemicals and "new" bacteria being discovered in our drinking water. KNOW WHAT'S IN YOUR WATER, PLEASE!

Anyway, when I got back to the airport for my return flight and reopened the book I'd begun reading, the very next chapter began with the admonishment to not stop dairy consumption suddenly, as it can precipitate very uncomfortable mucous production.

They could have put that as the last sentence in the prior chapter! It's worth repeating:

Never stop cow dairy cold turkey! Gradually taper off dairy to diminish the chances of a mucous overload.

Bottom line: Recognize the potential for food allergies, sensitivities, and/or intolerances. "One man's meat is another man's poison!" Rotate foods you *can* consume healthily, especially if you're a B blood type. Bored Bs are Bad Bs!

Drink Clean Water

How much do you weigh? Go check! I'll wait right here for you. In fact, jot that number down for easy reference later:

Weight _____ Date _____

Divide your weight (in pounds) into thirds. That's the minimal amount of water your body needs to function (in fluid ounces—jot it down on the next page).

Go back to your total weight and cut that number in half. That's the amount of water you need daily when you're active and/or sweating (jot that down below, too).

It's easy math. For example, if you weigh 120 pounds, your daily water consumption is 40-60 ounces.

If you weigh 150 pounds, you need 50-75 ounces of water every day. 180 pounds, 60-90 ounces of daily water intake.

What's your range? Feel free to use a calculator! I'll wait. In fact, I'll go to my measured-out pitcher of water for the day and pour a cup of that into the kettle to make some herbal tea....

Required amount of water each day:

_____

Your water needs to be *clean*. The Environmental Working Group offers a free Tap Water Database by zip code to determine what your municipally-treated water contains. Check that out. I've had patients/clients whose chief complaint cleared once their water situation was corrected.

They also offer recommendations for various water filtration needs. https://www.ewg.org/tapwater/

If you have a well, please send a sample of your water off annually for an assay. Some counties offer this service for free, or there might be a small fee. If your county does not offer this service, consider paying a reputable lab for a determination of what your water contains or hiring a reputable well-servicing company to inspect your well cap/cover, the lining, then the inner workings of the pump mechanism and the water itself. Well caps can grow interesting, yet unhealthy, organisms.

Knowing what is in your water helps inform your next decisions for filtration, if needed. I had a water guy install his proprietary, mineral-preserving reverse osmosis system in my crazy-cool house twenty years ago. After the Covid years, he quit the business and the other guys in town don't know what he used in his proprietary blend, so they use "stock" filters for reverse osmosis. Water expert Winston Kao has me concerned now about the lack of minerals and the presence of microplastics in my current set-up. I need to sell a lot of books to pay for the reconstruction of my spiral staircase and Winston's multi-vortex, mechanical water filtration system. (Thank you for your support!) His information is in References and Resources.

Now that you know how much to drink and how to get your water clean, let's talk about how to *drink* that volume of water over the course of your day.

Measure it out. It's simple. Get an attractive container that holds what you require and measure the minimal amount you need; mark it with a crayon. Then add water until you reach your maximal amount you would need on a very active day and mark it again. Aim to drink all of the water poured most days. Use this measured water for making green tea or herbal tisanes (the fancy and correct word for herbal "tea"), which count *toward* your water intake.

Beverages that count *against* your water intake include coffee, soda, black tea, and alcohol. For now, for each "negative" beverage, drink the same amount of "positive" beverage. If you're addicted to coffee or tea or alcohol, this will be a smart way to start diminishing your dependence on them while improving overall health. (Go, *you!*)

Feel free to guzzle first thing in the morning: eight, twelve, or even sixteen ounces of water. After that, sip on your water throughout the day, between meals. Have water with you at the table, but please don't drink too much of it just prior to eating. Keep your digestive acid aflame for optimal absorption of nutrients. Stop drinking water three hours before bedtime for better sleep outcomes.

Carry your water with you to work, school, and when you're driving around town. Glass is best for your water container, but glass containers are not welcome in pools or various sports venues due to the potential for breakage. Food grade stainless steel (18/8) is second best. Plastic bottles—especially the "squishy" kind—are not recommended, but drinking from them is arguably better than drinking no water at all.

Squishy (and many non-squishy) water bottles and baby bottles are made of bisphenol-A (BPA) plastic. Ten million tons of this stuff was estimated to have been produced in 2022 alone. It's flippin' *everywhere*!

BPA is a "persistent" (meaning it will never decompose completely) chemical. It has been implicated in the development of type 2 diabetes. It's also a xenoestrogen, meaning it mimics estrogen in humans but definitely isn't estrogen. It's an endocrine system disruptor. BPA can leach out of its boundaries and into the substance it's supposed to be holding, especially when warmed (when the plastic is softened). That means the water inside the plastic becomes plastic-infused water (*plastic tea?*), or the baby formula inside the plastic bottle becomes plastic-infused baby formula when heated.

This brings to mind the very kind people who keep cases of bottled water in the trunks of their cars to hand to the homeless. Think of the cases of bottled water stacked on tables sitting in the baking sunlight near hiking/biking trails for thirsty athletes. Imagine the warehouses that aren't climate-controlled storing cases of plastic-bottled water for our future purposes. All those plastic water bottles subjected to great heat end up containing plastic-infused water.

Even when we're trying to improve health, trying to improve society, trying to make things better all around us… there are obstacles to health. "My people perish for lack of knowledge." — Hosea 4:6"

I volunteered at a music festival last year and was asked to please bring a case of water to share. I brought a case of glass-bottled fizzy water. This year, I didn't volunteer, but I still went to the annual music festival and ran into a coworker volunteer from last year who remembered me because I'd brought in "bougie" water. "Bougie" as in "bourgeois" or "rich/wealthy." I wasn't showing off; I was diminishing our consumption of plastics that won't ever leave our system or this planet, but will leave a devastating mark on human and planetary health.

Checklist for Water Basics

- Drink _____ oz of water daily
- Water means water, green tea, and herbal tisanes
- Send out well-water sample for evaluation annually
- Test municipally-treated tap water (https://www.ewg.org/tapwater/)
- Get a water filter, if needed
- 18/8 stainless steel or glass water bottle to carry around

Advanced Topics Messages In Water

This one's always a fun conversation. Have you ever heard of quantum _____? (Quantum physics, quantum mechanics, quantum biology… ?) When Sir Isaac Newton blew our minds with his findings, we put his name on everything "new" for a while—Newtonian physics, Newtonian mechanics. His ideas helped form a conceptual framework for how the universe and all that is within it functions.

Welcome to the age of Quantum Theory! Remember reading about macrovascular and microvascular outcomes with the anti-diabetes medication? Newtonian and quantum understandings are a *little bit* like that, in that Newton's ideas about big concepts like gravity and objects in motion are deterministic inside our macroscopic world. Quantum thinking seems a bit mind-twisting in that it looks for probabilities in our microscopic world, where particles don't always act in ways one might expect. With this in mind, let's revisit the topic of water.

As you are aware, our planet is about 70 percent water, just like our bodies. As you also know, water is a most astonishing substance, serving humans in four different phases.

FOUR? I only know about three: solid ice, liquid water, and gaseous steam. What's the fourth phase of water?

Excellent set up for me, Reader—thank you! The fourth phase of water is gel. And if the brilliant Gerald Pollock, PhD researcher in water is correct, that's a phase water takes inside our blood vessels, creating current for flow as well as electrical current within and part of the flow. I'll wait while you read that again.

Isn't that so cool? The way medical students are currently being taught about the heart as a pump and how muscles contract and even what we extract from the air we breathe is all subject to change because of quantum theories and understanding the fourth phase of water!

Readers, as advanced as we Americans think we are, we're well behind when it comes to understanding the totality of humanness. Other world medicines (being rapidly replaced by our current petro-chemical disease-management model) understand that all our layers and pieces/parts are connected. Whatever goes into our ears as music alters our thinking and our emotions. What hurts our feelings can manifest as pain in the body.

How does that happen?

Through *water*, dear Reader! Water not only cleans our cells but also allows for communication inside the cell and between cells. Dirty water = dirty cells and dirty blood. Have you ever seen a pond in the south in late August? Funk, my friend, is all I can say about that. Until the cleansing rains return, things will be dying in that shrinking, funked-up pond. (As clean as the rain can be anymore, anyway.)

Conventional medicine doctors might have us believe that acupuncture is craziness, but when viewed through the quantum lens, it makes sense. Those meridians correspond to wider bands of fascia. Fascia is the connective tissue that holds our disparate parts together as one complete whole. Fascia is also the highway of water-based messaging. When observed, there is a measurable change in electrophysiology at meridian points.

Ooh! Measuring things we can't see is new! You're so right, Reader! Thanks for pointing that out.

Chinese medicine, Unani/Yunani medicine, Ayurvedic medicine, homeopathic medicine, Thai medicine, Japanese medicine (Kampo/Kanpo), Korean medicine (Hanyak, Hanbag), aboriginal medicine, European, Greco-Arab, and Islamic botanical medicines, and eclectic and folkloric medicines, all recognize our inherent interconnectedness. Not just our own pieces/parts with other of our own pieces/parts, but the interconnectedness of all things, microscopic and macroscopic, quantum and Newtonian!

Conventional medicine centers itself around prescription drugs and procedures.

How did that happen? It's a sad tale, Reader, but a worthy question. I'll provide a link to a ninety-minute documentary that explains just how healthcare became sick-care in America https://talknatural.com/documentary.html and leave the topic on this disturbing note: the root word from which we get our words pharmacy, pharmacology, pharmaceuticals, etc. is the Greek word, *pharmakeia*, which means witchcraft, magic, use of spells and potions, often involving drugs; in other words, *drug-related sorcery*.

Before one of you comes after me, remember that I can't make this stuff up! Also remember that I ride a motorcycle and would WANT heroic emergency medicine should there be a mishap on the highway involving me on that motorcycle. There is a time and place for most drugs in the market. But there is iatrogenesis/inherent harm built into drug use—prescription or otherwise.

Move Your Body

PLAY! Get up off the couch and dance! Climb a tree! Fly a kite! Go skating, biking, hiking, camping, swimming! Yes, you *could* join a gym. (Yes, you *should* hire a personal trainer!) Whatever you choose to do, make it enjoyable!

"It's fun to have fun, but you have to know how." — Dr. Seuss.

If you have forgotten how to play, can you remember what you used to love when you were a kid? Balance and agility permitting, do that activity now! You might have to work up to it but take the first step. Then the second. Before you know it, you'll be swimming a mile (for fun!) or bicycling seventy-five miles in a day just because you can and it feels good.

If you have **high blood pressure**, exercise of any kind helps your brain know that the dangerous "tiger" you've been perceiving has been dealt with appropriately. You might want to consider kickboxing. Or, just kick a box. Grab an empty cardboard box, tape or fold it shut, and give it a good kick outside. The sound and the action can be very satisfying. After you've kicked the box to smithereens, simply gather the pieces and place them in the recycle bin. Ah!

If you have **dyslipidemia**, just do something that's *fun*! People with cholesterol abnormalities often feel constrained, held back, slightly irritated, and frustrated with a life circumstance—it might be their job, relationship, or living environment. Simply moving in an enjoyable way throws off much of those stress-related hormones, allowing for decompression in your psyche, resulting in less overall inflammation. Try it!

If you have **type 2 diabetes**, take a brisk twenty-minute walk right after your largest meal of the day. Don't even do the dishes first! Refrigerate the left-overs, put your walking shoes on, and *go*! This helps make your insulin receptors more receptive, drawing available insulin into the cells and normalizing blood glucose.

Struggling with weight? Start walking. Work up to walking at 65 percent of your maximum heart rate for about forty-five minutes. Do this six days a week for the most effective, efficient weight loss. (*What?* Move it or lose it, my dear Reader. I want you to keep your toes, your feet, your lower legs, your ability to ambulate! The final choice is, as always, *yours*.) Determine your max heart rate with this equation:

$$[220 - \text{Age (years)}] \times 0.65 = \text{targeted heart beats per minute}$$

Get Radically Restorative Sleep

Who here has heard about "sleep hygiene?" I hadn't either until naturopathic medical school! Let me tell you about it.

Sleep is the primary space/time when we heal. We can only heal when our bodies are in parasympathetic nervous system dominance, and sleep is when we're in that state for the longest period of time. Roughly a third of our lives is spent sleeping! Cats sleep about 90 percent of their lives. No wonder they get nine lives! (No, cats don't *really* live nine lives. I saw a T-shirt once that read, "Every good life has room for nine cats." Number 7 is with me now.)

In order to ensure we get the proper restorative rest from our nightly slumber, here are the sleep hygiene rules:

- Your bedroom should be several degrees cooler than the rest of the house
- The bedroom should be darker than the rest of the house (use light blocking curtains, if necessary)
- The bedroom should be reserved for sex and sleep. Reading is allowed, preferably paper media.
- No electronics in the bedroom: TV, computer, cell phone, regular land-line phone, iPads/tablets, and gaming devices should be left outside the bedroom. In fact, all electronics should be turned *off* three hours prior to bedtime so that your mid/hind brain takes a break from reactivity, allowing your mind to subsequently settle down.
- No food or drink for three hours prior to bedtime, so that you're resting, not digesting, and to keep you from experiencing multiple trips to the bathroom.
- The "sweet spot" for healing is to be in bed with the lights off by ten p.m.

The pushback I receive when discussing sleep hygiene still surprises me. Reader, you're here because you want something better for yourself, right? That means you must change the habits that got you into your current predicament. How are your current "bad" habits serving you? What's keeping you from engaging in health-promoting new habits?

If you've not done the various exercises assigned or made new habits from each section of instruction above, Reader, stop here, please. You aren't quite ready for what's coming up. Go back to the unfinished work and complete that so you'll be prepared for this section. Remember, we've been laying a foundation for health and success. I don't want you derailed before you get started.

If you have done all the exercises, move forward with me now.

Monitor your objective signs and subjective symptoms all along the way!

Take pictures!

Delving Into The Immaterial Aspects Of Yourself: Emotions-Mind-Spirit

Live Life On Purpose

Does the work you do light you up? Does it feed your soul? If money weren't a consideration, what would you *choose* to do? Why? Whom would you *choose* to serve? Why?

These are not rhetorical questions. Please answer.

_____

_____

_____

_____

Overworking can cause **type 2 diabetes and obesity**. Unrelenting stress can cause high **blood pressure**. Or stress can look more like inflammation, which is the working theory now for what causes **high cholesterol levels**.

Once you get clear on what you want, start pursuing that path. It's never too late! I was a pharmacist for a decade before deciding to quit my career, sell everything we owned, leave everyone we knew, to move across the universe so I could go back to school full-time to become a naturopathic physician. My newlywed spouse thought I'd lost my mind, but it worked out!

Make Relationships Healthy Again

Despite my own and others' objections to this, humans were designed to live in community with other humans. Some of us have a greater capacity for greater numbers of other humans in our community, and others need a smaller community in sub-sets. Some of us have only one or two others who have earned the right and honor to contact our inner selves. There's no wrong answer except the misconception that "I can do life on my own."

Early in my naturopathic career, I had a client travel a considerable distance to my office for guidance about his *uncontrolled blood pressure*. He'd tried an agent from every class of anti-hypertensive medications on the market, but they all stopped working in a matter of weeks. He'd also tried multiple diets, to no lasting effect. In his mid-fifties, he was in middle management, in the midst of a difficult marriage, and estranged from both of his adult sons. He was afraid of dying young, as his father and uncles had. He believed high blood pressure was in his genes because of the family history.

Honestly, y'all, he'd tried so many things, and I was so new to being a practitioner, I was at a loss about how to proceed. To calm my own nerves, I suggested body work in the form of cranio-sacral therapy. He complied and lay on my treatment table, his wife seated in the room with us.

Have you ever sensed trouble when entering a room or picked up on another's emotional state when they are nearby? That happened. With one of my hands under his back and the other over his heart, I heard my voice ask, "Do you give love well? Do you receive love well? How are you with forgiveness?" He began to shake on the table as his wife began to sob. Then he got off the table. And he was *mad!* With trembling of my own, I moved over and sat next to his wife.

"What did you *do* to me?" he demanded.

Before this starts to read like fiction, let me just tell you what happened. His wife let me know about the estranged kids and the state of their marriage—they'd already started the conversation about divorce after nearly thirty years together. He had been estranged from his father. Work was a mess and he blamed everyone but himself for why he hadn't been promoted. In short, he was an angry man. A hard-hearted man.

The metaphorical state of our being often shows up in a very physical way.

I offered other therapies including forgiveness work. We talked about his belief system. He began to see his own incongruent behavior. I prescribed a diet specific to him, which he tried with more success than prior diets. What he experienced through our conversations was a heart change. And his blood pressure normalized. About a year later, he was mending bridges with his sons, his marriage was back on track, and he was looking for a more meaningful job.

Heart issues are where I typically use a select few botanicals to help with forgiveness and old metaphorical heart wounds. It's less about what therapy I choose and more about *why* I pick them. If we go back to the Therapeutic Order and Lindlahr's six pillars of health, this particular client needed help on Step 2, Lindlahr 6.

Step 2: Stimulate the *Vis!* One of the principles of naturopathic medicine is *Vis Medicatrix Naturae,* Latin for "the healing power of nature." Some would argue that the meaning is merely speaking of using natural agents. Others say this is far deeper and more mysterious, referencing that which enlivens our very being. I really like Henry Lindlahr's definition in his 6th pillar: "Arouse the individual to the highest possible degree to the consciousness of personal accountability and the necessity of intelligent personal effort and self-help."

To "arouse an individual" means to wake him up. "To the highest possible degree" means as much as she is able. "To the consciousness of personal accountability" means awareness and responsibility of your own actions and how they impact others. "And the necessity of intelligent personal effort and self-help" means understanding he's got a brilliant mind and an amazing body for which only he is ultimately responsible!

I'm a fan of asking my clients with chronic disease why they think their bodies picked that issue to get their attention. So…

Those of you with **high blood pressure**—what similarities or differences do you share with my hard-hearted client? How well do *you* give and receive love? How well do you give and receive forgiveness? If your spirit were trying to get a message through your heart to you, what might that message be?

_____

_____

_____

_____

If your **cholesterol** is out of whack, how can you get curious about systemic inflammation? Where are you feeling constrained? What's frustrating you? What's irritating? How do you feel "trapped"?

_____

_____

_____

_____

For the **diabetic**, where's the sweetness in your life? What makes your life lovely? What do you want more of?

_____

_____

_____

_____

Sometimes, when we're curious enough, we can get all the answers we need to make the changes necessary to cure ourselves.

Non-edible Consumptions

We consume many things other than food and drink—things like music, movies, books, magazines, and social media. These contribute to or detract from vibrant health. They also impact our thoughts, emotions, and behaviors also.

This family loves music! From a very early age, I played piano; my boys also loved music early on and tried their skills at clarinet, flute, drums, guitar, and piano. When I take breaks from working, I typically have music playing.

Before we drove across the country, one son asked me which artists and albums I wanted included in my portion of our combined playlist. I told him. While driving, with me singing along, he started shaking his head. "Mom, I cannot *believe* you listen to this. After the talks we've had about lyrics? This stuff is trash!" He was right!

When the kids were younger, we homeschooled them. I chose their curriculum, their activities, their music, movies, books, and their friends. It was great! :-)

One day, the younger son came bopping into the house singing along with the catchy tune that was playing only in his head. He's always had a sense for music, so I could readily identify the song he was singing—but who had played *that* song in the hearing of my child?

I stopped him in his tracks to ask, "Honey-child, what are you singing to yourself?"

To which he replied with great exuberance, "A *song*, Momma!"

"Yes, I know you're singing a song, Sweets. What is that song—and your voice—saying to you?"

He paused for a moment and thought about the words before answering: "I'm a loser, baby, so why don't you kill me." (Mic drop.)

I know that song! It is catchy—and disturbing!

I did the same "quiz game" with the older son as a teen. By then, he was no longer homeschooled and no longer allowing me to choose his friends and music. He was regularly exposed to the whims and often destructive nature of our culture—and I caught him singing a song that I knew would embarrass the tar out of him if he only thought about it for a split second. Which he did. And he was.

Readers, we all do this! We are like sponges, soaking up what's in our environment—the good, the bad, and the downright ugly. Don't soak up trash, friends.

If you want vibrant health, start taking inventory of *all.the.things!* What are you listening to in the car? What are you reading before bed? Which movies, concerts, theater productions do you attend? Which thoughts continually play in the circuitous route of your mind? How many hours do you spend daily scrolling through other people's lives on social media?

Seriously! Write down the answers.

I've known and worked with folks whose favorite TV-show personalities and book characters were more alive than the family members living under the same roof with them. I love books! (I'm writing one right now.) But they shouldn't take the place of those you say you love.

On a stay at someone else's house, I saw a piece of art with the ocean as the background picture and these words superimposed:

"Emotions are like waves, they come and go. We decide which ones we surf."

Get curious about why you choose the things you choose. Choose those things that bring you life, move you toward health, and keep you aligned with your purpose!

Have You Lost Yourself Along The Way? Trauma Timeline Revisited.

When you were writing out your own Trauma Timeline, what emotions came up for you? Who taught you about emotions? What did your family model for you and/or demand from you when it came to emotions?

_____

_____

_____

_____

If we had to, we could put all the emotions into four major categories: Glad, Mad, Sad and Bad. Fortunately, others have written books that help us differentiate the nuances of various experiences and emotions, my favorites being works by Karla McLaren, Brene Brown, and Emily McMason (online workbooks). There's a useful "emotional ladder" floating around the interwebs that looks like this (by Abraham Hicks. I don't know what you know about Abraham Hicks, so I'll just say: Don't throw the baby out with the bathwater):

1. Joy/Appreciation/Empowerment/Freedom/Love
2. Passion
3. Enthusiasm/Eagerness/Happiness
4. Positive Expectation/Belief
5. Optimism
6. Hopefulness
7. Contentment
8. Boredom
9. Pessimism
10. Frustration/Irritation/Impatience
11. Overwhelm

12. Disappointment
13. Doubt
14. Worry
15. Blame
16. Discouragement
17. Anger
18. Revenge
19. Hatred/Rage
20. Jealousy
21. Insecurity/Guilt/Unworthiness
22. Fear/Grief/Desperation/Despair/Powerlessness

The reason I like this is that it encourages those living amid the bottom rungs to aspire to the next rung up, rather than the top of the ladder. We don't typically drop from Joy to Despair in one fell swoop—just like we don't go from vibrant wellness to grave illness overnight. "Chronic" denotes a timeline—so it's reasonable to set expectations when we find ourselves at the bottom of the emotional ladder that we will be able to climb upward again, not catapult to the top.

If you experienced complex childhood trauma, or you have a high ACE (Adverse Childhood Events) score, or because of drug use (prescription or not) you've experienced dissociation, please find a counselor with experience in dissociative disorders. You'll need to create safe space for healing and learn to stay in your body while recalling painful memories and naming emotions. When you can recall the painful memory, feel the emotion it provoked, and name the emotion, all while staying inside your body—no spirit/soul hanging out in the ceiling corner—you'll be well on your way to healthy wholeness.

It's been a hot minute since we did any exercises, Reader, so let's *go!* Answer these questions for the sake of your healthier self:

Who do you want to be?

_____
_____
_____
_____

What do you want to *do?*

_____
_____
_____

Where would you like to be, doing what you want to do?

_____
_____
_____
_____

When you pass from this realm of existence, what are you hoping will be said about you?

_____
_____
_____
_____

How are you living your eulogy now?

_____
_____
_____
_____

To help with those questions, go back to Exercise 3 at the beginning of this portion of the book. Read over your answers. Now add to it your self-inventory of the gifts, talents, skills, education, and experiences that have shaped you.

Gifts:

_____
_____
_____
_____

Talents:

_____
_____
_____
_____

Skills:

_____
_____
_____
_____

Education:

_____
_____
_____
_____

Experiences:

_____
_____
_____
_____

If you need help with this, ask a small handful of your best friends who know you in various settings to tell you who you are. This is called the Fishbowl Exercise or Goldfish Exercise, as if you're a goldfish in the fishbowl on display for all to see. You're inviting trusted people to give you a glimpse of who you are through their less biased-about-you lenses.

Add in the following, Reader:

What legacy did your family of origin leave you? (This could, potentially, be specific things you intend to demolish as you make changes in your lifestyle, leaving a new and very different legacy for your children.)

_____
_____
_____
_____

What are your desires? Maybe you've never spoken them aloud before, so writing them here may feel reckless, even dangerous. Do so now, if you dare.

Disease Reversal: Hypertension, Dyslipidemia, Type 2 Diabetes

_____
_____
_____
_____

What do other people tell you about yourself that you take for granted, because you assume (careful!) that everyone has that particular skill or talent or ability? (This is probably your personal "superpower!")

_____
_____
_____
_____

Finally, what's your personal mantra? Do you have a verse from Scripture that guides you, or a snippet from a poem that speaks to you? Jot that down here.

_____
_____
_____
_____

Nice work, Reader! Are you starting to get a feel for your life's purpose, that it's something much bigger than what you could accomplish on your own, that you're here to thrive rather than just survive? You *matter*, Reader! Who'd now choose to keep on keepin' on in chronic dis-ease with all this powerful information? We're on the cusp of Disease Reversal, my friend!

How To Talk To Prescribers About De-Prescribing The Drugs

Whoo-hoo! You've made it here!

At this point, maybe you've already started to use some of this information to change your habits and your life. If you have, you might be noticing a decrease in your numbers, whether that's blood pressure, cholesterol, or blood glucose. Good job, Reader! I may have to start calling you a "Reversal-er!" Isn't it *so* fun to e-s-r-e-v-e-r (that's "reverse" spelled in reverse) chronic disease? Especially when your own doctor says it can't be done? ☺

Ok. If you've done the work and you're already seeing your desired results, it's time to gather your logs of numbers proving, objectively, that you've made sufficient changes to warrant drug reduction or removal. Be prepared to tell your prescriber what you've done differently and how you subjectively feel: weak and woozy or lightheaded when moving quickly from lying down to sitting up or from sitting to standing (**blood pressure**); increased muscle aches/pain, decreased interest in sex, foggy thinking (**cholesterol**—although your lifestyle changes may very well prevent these symptoms from occurring); feeling shaky, increased irritability, mood swings returning when they'd been dropping off (**diabetes**).

The combination of your objective numbers and subjective storyline might just be too compelling for a medical doctor to *not* reduce or remove a medication!

DON'T TAKE YOURSELF OFF PRESCRIPTION MEDICINES! If your prescriber won't listen to you, fire him and hire one that will work with you as part of your team. This is *your* health, after all!

Because conventional medicine is the source of information for Artificial Intelligence, and conventional medicine practitioners are not in the habit of de-prescribing—nor are they trained in de-prescribing—it can actually be dangerous to consult Artificial Intelligence about de-prescribing!

Find a doctor here to help you reduce/remove medication: https://naturopathicmedicineinstitute.org/

I've taught many of these doctors and they all know how to contact me, if necessary.

Did that wrap up too neatly? If you've been doing the exercises and putting into practical application the new information laid out in this book, Reader, I absolutely expect you to be ready for medication reduction and/or removal! There is *more to read, however…*

About A.M., to whom this book is dedicated

This book is dedicated posthumously to a man who was in his mid-sixties when we met, semi-retired from the police department after having served in the military in Vietnam. His wife was a client of mine—dear, sweet, kind, soft-spoken. He was the proverbial bull in the China shop—loud, irascible, stubborn. "The Wife" *made* him see me. He was carrying about forty pounds of extra weight along with the diagnoses of hypertension, dyslipidemia and—you guessed it!—type 2 diabetes. He wanted nothing to do with my dietary recommendations. He liked his steak "black and blue," his starchy potatoes, his excessive coffee consumption, and his *way!*

Something came over me amid his swagger and bluster, so I called him on it, making it sound like my recommendations—vegetarian fare with whole grains and wild-caught, cold-water fish—would be too difficult for him to follow. He rose immediately to the challenge. I scheduled him for follow-up six weeks later. Before he left my office that day, though, he drew a sketch of how my office should be arranged. Who knew he'd have talents in *feng shui*?

My workspace was a single-room office in those days with a desk, some bookshelves, other shelves with supplements, a filing cabinet, a treatment table, and a couple of chairs. His complaint about my office intrigued me, and his sketch made pretty good sense. I made the changes he recommended.

He arrived a few minutes early for his appointment, poked his head into my office, looked around with a satisfied grin and declared three things:

- That I was trainable; therefore…
- He'd be my new office manager, because…
- I'd done more for him in six weeks than his medical doctor had done in fourteen years.

He was a different man! And he proved to be the best volunteer office manager I've ever had. I miss him. He'd be quite proud of this book.

Final Remarks to Followers of YHWH

You may be among the most difficult to encourage to live more healthily. In my opinion, due to years of observation, God's church seems to have divorced healing (God's "impossible" work) from health (man's practical responsibility).

What?

Did I surprise you, Reader?

Yeah! Oh, wait. Is it the donut board? Hahaha! It's the donut board! Or... the anniversary lunch with food truck options? Wait! The Welcome or New Member Lunch/Supper with only in-house options? The small group fair with sodas and ice cream. Pizza brought in for the hospitality training. The Ministry Team Room snacks that wouldn't pass the "read the label out loud" test. Yikes! Splenda and NutraSweet and multiple-ingredient creamer in single-use plastic containers that have eternal shelf life and never require refrigeration! Keurig coffee in pods that will never decompose. Oh, my God! When did we quit being stewards of God's resources—including the gift God has given us called our bodies, which were made in His very image?

Wow, Reader—you nailed it! Need I say more?

Whenever Jesus got angry—and He most definitely got angry!—His anger was centered on the religious traditions of the day, like the hard-heartedness of those who were leaders of the Jewish people and the creation of rules to protect the rules so no one would break the rules, while altogether leaving out the *reason* for the rules.

The other day, my beloved husband was so busy doing things *for* me that he left no room for *me*.

That's how religion had become. So Jesus left Heaven—the Creator became like the created—to straighten out the mess, showing His disciples (and subsequently us) how to live in His Kingdom right here on Earth. And it just didn't make sense to most of the people watching.

God said to His prophet, Hosea, "My people perish for lack of knowledge!" Truly, even though Jesus came to Earth Himself to teach us to love one another, to live altogether differently, and to leave us with His own Spirit for comfort and counsel (fulfilling all the Law of the Old Testament that God had laid out for His people in His plan of redemption, allowing sinful humans to abide in His holy Presence)—*we still aren't getting it right!*

Case in point: Christ-followers have no better statistics than non-Christ-followers in rates of obesity, hypertension, cholesterol abnormalities, type 2 diabetes; cancer, autoimmune disorders... *disease* of any kind! Nor do lovers of Jesus have better statistics than haters in rates of abortion, suicide, bankruptcy, addiction, or divorce.

How are we to be a *light* to this darkening world when we're as dim as the rest?

I am *not at all* suggesting that your salvation is in question while you drink that milk shake, Reader. I *am* suggesting that, if you proclaim Jesus as your Savior—that's a free gift to all; if you proclaim Jesus as your LORD, KING, GOD—that costs *everything!* Your body. Your emotions. Your mind. Your spirit. Your finances. Your dreams. Your marriage. Your children. Your choices. Your lifestyle.

The gifts, talents, skills, education, experiences, desires—*all that you are and have* that was mercifully granted to you by GOD Almighty—is ultimately His. That's what the LORD of lords, KING of kings, GOD of gods requires.

Gulp.

Remember when the Pharisees were trying to trip Jesus up about paying taxes to Rome? Mark 12:13-17 (Matthew gives his account, too, 22:20-21):

> "13 Later they sent some of the Pharisees and Herodians to Jesus to catch him in his words. 14 They came to him and said, "Teacher, we know that you are a man of integrity. You aren't swayed by others, because you pay no attention to who they are; but you teach the way of God in accordance with the truth. Is it right to pay the imperial tax to Caesar or not? 15 Should we pay or shouldn't we?"
>
> But Jesus knew their hypocrisy. "Why are you trying to trap me?" he asked. "Bring me a denarius and let me look at it." 16 They brought the coin, and he asked them, "Whose image is this? And whose inscription?"
>
> "Caesar's," they replied.
>
> 17 Then Jesus said to them, "Give back to Caesar what is Caesar's and to God what is God's."
>
> And they were amazed at him.

Why were they amazed? Because *they understood what He was saying!* Which is...

We are made in the very image of God. He bought us with the cost of His perfect Son, Jesus. We owe Him EVERYTHING: body, emotions, will, mind, soul, spirit, work, finances, relationships. The free gift of Jesus demands our all. If we profess that we follow His Son, Jesus Christ, His inscription (blood) is on us! Better still that we GIVE Him EVERYTHING out of the sheer desperation of humanity and as being the living sacrifice He calls us to be, working in cooperative interdependence with Him in all things!

Final Remarks to Followers of YHWH

This is what God says about our bodies:

- "Don't you know that you yourselves are God's temple and that God's Spirit lives in you? If anyone destroys God's temple, God will destroy him; for God's temple is sacred, and you are that temple." — I Corinthians 3:16-17
- "Do you not know that your body is a temple of the Holy spirit, who is in you, whom you have received from God? You are not your own; you were bought at a price. Therefore, honor God with your body." — I Corinthians 6:19-20
- "What agreement is there between the temple of God and idols? For we are the temple of the living God." — II Corinthians 6:16 ("Idols" are anything you have in a higher priority than your KING, Jesus.)
- "Therefore, I urge you, brothers, in view of God's mercy, to offer your bodies as living sacrifices, holy and pleasing to God—this is your spiritual act of worship. Do not conform any longer to the pattern of this world but be transformed by the renewing of your mind. Then you will be able to test and approve what God's will is—His good, pleasing and perfect will." — Romans 12:1-2 (Body, Mind, Spirit!)
- "Does the Lord delight in burnt offerings and sacrifices as much as in obeying the voice of the Lord? To obey is better than sacrifice, and to heed is better than the fat of rams." — I Samuel 15:22 (Will, Emotions!)

God also tells us what we can expect if/when we *don't* responsibly take care of what's been entrusted to us:

- "To one he gave five talents of money, to another two talents, and to another one talent, each according to his ability....
- "... Take the talent from him and give it to the one who has the ten talents. For everyone who has will be given more, and he will have an abundance. Whoever does not have, even what he has will be taken from him. And throw that worthless servant outside, into the darkness, where there will be weeping and gnashing of teeth.'" — Matthew 25:15-30

Commands concerning foods (Deuteronomy) were

- To set the Israelites apart—"Out of all the peoples on the face of the earth, the Lord has chosen you to be his treasured possession."
- To allow for long life in the land they were about to be given. (We know now that those who consume pork and/or shellfish as dietary staples have worse outcomes in the event of an epidemic.)
- The commands went so far as to specify male circumcision for God's chosen people, to set them apart by physical appearance.

And all the bacon lovers ask, *"What about Peter's vision?"* Fortunately, Peter interpreted his dream for us:

- "Again a voice came to him a second time, 'What God has cleansed, no longer consider unholy.'"

  "And he (Peter, explaining the vision) said to them, 'You yourselves know how unlawful it is for a man who is a Jew to associate with a foreigner or to visit him; and yet God has shown me that I should not call any man unholy or unclean.'" — Acts 10:15 and Acts 11:28

Peter is accused of eating unclean food, then explains why (and how) God allowed this. Through the whole passage, we see that Peter ate what was for the gain of the gospel, for the salvation of others. It does not say that he ate whatever he wanted to. — Acts 11:3

In other words, these passages explain the reason for eating otherwise "unclean" things is the salvation of others, not the satisfaction of your tongue.

- "'Everything is permissible'—but not everything is beneficial. 'Everything is permissible'—but not everything is constructive. …So whether you eat or drink or whatever you do, do it all for the glory of God…so that they may be saved." — 1 Corinthians 10:23-33
- All things are lawful for me, but not all things are profitable. All things are lawful for me, but I will not be mastered by anything. — 1 Corinthians 6:12
- "Do not be overcome by evil, but overcome evil with good." — Romans 12:21

Choosing to eat something good—healthy, nutritious, beneficial—is showing respect for your physical body and the God who has lavished such a gift on you.

- "Therefore, to one who knows the right thing to do and does not do it, to him it is sin." — James 4:17

Ignorance may be bliss, but it'll still kill you! And *you*, Reader, are no longer ignorant!

- "Do not put out the Spirit's fire; do not treat prophecies with contempt. ***Test everything***. Hold on to the good. Avoid every kind of evil. May God himself, the God of peace, sanctify you through and through. May your whole spirit, soul and body be kept blameless at the coming of our Lord Jesus Christ. The One who calls you is faithful and He will do it." — I Thessalonians 5:19-24
- "Finally, brethren, whatever is true, whatever is honorable, whatever is right, whatever is pure, whatever is lovely, whatever is of good repute, if there is any excellence and if anything worthy of praise, dwell on these things." — Philippians 4:8

Remember all those verses in the Bible about guarding the tongue? Rightly, we need to mind what comes out of our mouths, choosing to speak LIFE to the other body-wrapped spirits with whom we come into contact. Look how much trouble the tongue gets us into with food! Every good thing God has given has been met with a deceptive substitute by the Adversary. Eve was tempted with *food*. She failed the test. Jesus was tempted with food. He passed! Why would we think we'd be "safe" from food-based temptations? We're not!

Let your mind dwell on what is lovely and pure and worthy of praise, instead of dwelling on wanting to eat, eating unconsciously, or eating for comfort; scrolling through social media endlessly; or listening/watching things that would make you squirm if a close relative were right there with you.

Drawing again on wisdom from my pastor, who is diligently encouraging us all to *grow* as present-day disciples/"first followers" of Jesus, you are STACKED for a life on purpose:

- *S* **cripture**. What words guide you? What verse or passage really "speaks" to you, personally and powerfully? There's a reason for that!
- *T* **eam**. Surround yourself with a community of people who are different enough to continually teach you and similar enough to hold you steady on your God-appointed adventure.
- *A* **ptitude**. Use your "superpowers" for good in this life!
- *C* **alling**. What is it that pesters you? What desires or directions feel like a tug on your heart, mind and life? What and who are calling you to serve?
- *K* **in**. Yep, family. We inherit the good and the bad. Sometimes we need to break an unhealthy cycle; sometimes we need to continue the good trend that was started in previous generations. Usually, it's a combination of both.
- *E* **xperiences**. Without my pharmacy experience and my Job-experience (and my Jonah-experience and my Mary-and-Martha-experience), this book would never have happened. Everything happens for a reason.
- *D* **ependency**. If your dream is attainable in your own strength, I'm going to suggest you're not dreaming big enough. (*Circle Maker*, Mark Batterson.) A few years ago, I was challenged to up my game from walking with 100,000 people through their disease-reversal processes to 1,000,000. God is bigger than your dreams. Aim for "cooperative interdependence" with Him to partner for *His* dreams to become your reality! (*Royal Partners*, Larry Fox.)

But what if I was born crippled? What if I suffered an accident that has greatly limited my physical capacity?

Great questions, Reader! First, this book is talking about *lifestyle-driven diseases*. Others who have been in accidents—and other life-altering experiences—have written their stories in books. I'm thinking about Joni Erickson-Tada, Anne Frank, Harriet Tubman, and Louis Braille. I don't believe there is any such thing as an "accident" and God surely doesn't make mistakes. Still, we live in a broken world where bad things happen to good people. Paul told us in his letter to the Roman church that "in all things God works for the good of those who love him, who have been called according to his purpose." — Romans 8:28.

Many people who were born with disabilities have done great things for God and their fellow man! Helen Keller, Nick Vujicic, and Andrea Bocelli come to mind. God's not looking for perfection in the people He chooses to partner with Him; He's looking for willingness to leave our own wills in obedience to following His will. Closer to home for me is a powerfully gifted woman in my church who was born with cerebral palsy and is a great role model because of her devotion to God!

Do what is in your power as an expression of gratitude to your Maker—that's health. Rely on Him to do the impossible—that's healing. This is an example of cooperative interdependence!

Turn your STACKED life given by God back over to God. Ask that He make the best use of all He's given. Be ready to *do*, Reader! God is not tame. He is not to be put in the position of a personal assistant.

One more passage of Scripture, repeated from above, in its larger context. This is Paul speaking to the Christians in Rome about the Jewish people breaking God's Laws to the point of being dispersed across the nations, which brought about God's long-range plan of redemption, including for us Gentiles. After the history lesson, this is what Paul writes:

Oh, the depth of the riches of the wisdom and knowledge of God!

> How unsearchable his judgments,
>
> and his paths beyond tracing out!

34 Who has known the mind of the Lord?

> Or who has been his counselor?

35 Who has ever given to God,

> that God should repay them?

36 For from Him and through Him and for Him are all things.

> To Him be the glory forever! Amen.

Therefore, I urge you, brothers and sisters, in view of God's mercy, to offer your bodies as a living sacrifice, holy and pleasing to God—this is your true and proper worship. — Romans 11:33-36 through 12:1

You know what the *big* difference is about being a living sacrifice, as opposed to a dead one, Reader? It's your *choice* to stay on the altar—to do what God has purposed for you to do, faithfully stewarding all that He has given to you, including your health—or crawl right off that altar to do your own thing. Free choice, Reader. Free will.

{sigh.}

I'm a lover of good books. I hope you've found something "good" within these pages. One of my favorite series is *The Chronicles of Narnia*, by C.S. Lewis. I'll end the first book in this series with a passage from the first book in that series.

"Who is Aslan?" asked Susan.

"Aslan?" said Mr. Beaver. "Why don't you know? He's the King. . . .

"Is—is he a man?" asked Lucy.

"Aslan a man!" said Mr. Beaver sternly. "Certainly not. I tell you he is the King of the wood and the son of the great Emperor-Beyond-the-Sea. Don't you know who is the King of Beasts? Aslan is a lion—the Lion, the great Lion."

"Ooh!" said Susan. "I'd thought he was a man. Is he—quite safe?"

"Safe?" said Mr. Beaver.... Who said anything about safe? 'Course he isn't safe. But he's good. He's the King, I tell you."

    — Mr. Beaver to the Pevensie children in *The Lion, the Witch, and the Wardrobe*, by C.S. Lewis.

Wishing you WELL,

Christie Fleetwood, ND, RPh, FNMI, cBC

References and Resources

Books and lectures I used in the making of this book, in no particular order:

Nutritional Medicine, Alan Gaby

Herb, Nutrient and Drug Interactions, Mitchel Stargrove, et.al.

Medical Nutrition from Marz, Russell Marz

Blood Chemistry and CBC Analysis, Dicken Weatherby & Scott Ferguson

The Language of Emotions, Karla McLaren, https://karlamclaren.com/

Atlas of the Heart, Brene Brown (and several of her Ted Talks)

Women's Bodies, Women's Wisdom, Christiane Northrup

Anatomy of the Spirit, Caroline Myss

"Return to Me" worksheets, Emily McMason, https://emilymcmason.com/consulting/

The Body Keeps the Score, Bessel van der Kolk

https://www.drugs.com/pro/ and individual drug websites (every branded product has its very own!)

A Consumer's Dictionary of Food Additives, by Ruth Winters

TedMed "How Childhood Trauma Affects Health Across the Lifetime", Nadine Burke Harris

Health Psychology class paper on Dissociative Identity Disorder, best practices, Nicolas Hampton

Freedom in Christ, Neil T Anderson and Steve Goss

Leadership Pain, Samuel Chand

Classes at Cornerstone Assembly of God Church, North Chesterfield, VA

Royal Partners, Larry Fox

The Divine Conspiracy, Dallas Willard

Rare Earths: Forbidden Cures, by Joel Wallach and Ma Lan

Aristo Vojdani's research in autoimmunity and the role of gluten and cow proteins; presentation given at the American Association of Naturopathic Physicians, 2014(ish).

Winston Kao: https://winstonkao.com/, https://refreshingcleanwater.com/about-us/

Gerald Pollock's presentations at the Naturopathic Medicine Institute's Vital Gathering on the four phases of water (2023) and muscle contraction (2024).

Rick Kirschner's documentary, *How Healthcare Became Sickcare: the True History of Medicine*": https://talknatural.com/documentary.html

Healing is Voltage, by Jerry Tennant

Holistic Counseling: Introducing the Vis *Dialogue*, by Moshe Block

Nature Cure, by Henry Lindlahr

More than thirty-five years in the Healing Arts, listening to people's stories, researching and presenting on iatrogenesis ("diseases of the drugs") and what to do about it (informed consent and disease reversal)

And for you to print out and display prominently on your refrigerator, dear Reader, the one-page version of much of the homework around removing obstacles to cure and restoring (or establishing for the first time) the determinants of health. "Naturopathic Basics":

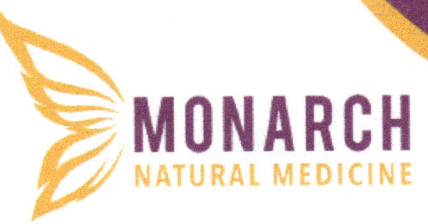

Naturopathic Basics

- Read labels! Avoid hydrogenated oils, trans fats, chemical sugar substitutes (Splenda, Nutrasweet, Equal), nitrites/nitrates, artificial ingredients, high fructose corn syrup, sodium benzoate, and anything you cannot pronounce. Topically, avoid sodium lauryl/laureth sulfates, parabens, petrolatum, mineral oil, aluminum.
- Adopt a whole foods diet, organic when possible, locally grown in season.
- Aim for 5 different vegetables and 2 fruits daily, mixed colors. Red, orange, yellow, green, blue, purple, and black (olives, berries, currants, grapes).
- Consume grass-pastured beef only, if you eat beef.
- Easier places to shop: Farmers' Markets, community supported agriculture groups (CSAs); local health food stores (Ellwood-Thompson's, Good Food Grocer); Whole Foods, Trader Joe's; "natural foods" sections in Kroger, Safeway, WalMart, Costco, etc.
- Recognize potential for food allergies/intolerances. One man's meat is another man's poison! Rotate foods you *can* consume healthily.
- Avoid microwave use.
- Sleep! The body can only repair while in parasympathetic nervous system dominance.
- Drink filtered water—1/3 to ½ your body weight in fluid ounces—daily. Green/herbal teas and coconut/cactus waters count!
- Exercise daily! Move your body every day, rain or shine, inside or outside. "Start low, go slow."
- Everything is connected to everything else--what impacts one area of your life will, to some degree, impact other parts of your life.
- List top 4 priorities in life. Does your lifestyle reflect those, in that order? If not, what steps need to be taken to truly walk your talk?